HELPING
CANCER PATIENTS
— EFFECTIVELY

HELPING CANCER PATIENTS — EFFECTIVELY

Nursing77 Books
Intermed Communications
Horsham, Pennsylvania

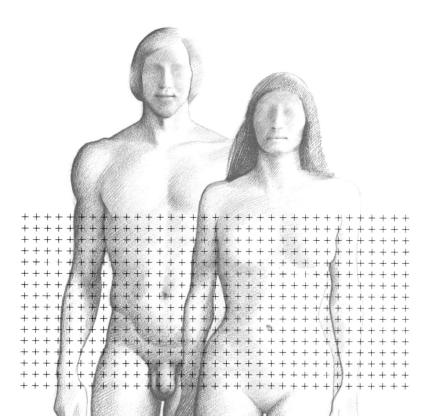

NURSING77 BOOKS
PUBLISHER: Eugene W. Jackson
Editorial Director: Daniel L. Cheney
Clinical Director: Margaret Van Meter, RN
Graphics Director: John Isely
Business Manager: Tom Temple

NURSING77 SKILLBOOK SERIES
MANAGING EDITOR: Patricia S. Chaney
Clinical Editor: Barbara McVan, RN
Book Editor: Jean Robinson
Marginalia Editor: Avery Rome
Copy Editor: Patricia A. Hamilton
Production Manager: Bernard Haas
Production Assistants: David C. Kosten, Margie Tyson
Designer: Maggie Arnott
Artists: Richard Oden, Robert Arufo, Robert Renn, Elizabeth Clark,
Sandra Simms, and Owen Heinrich
Cover and divider illustrations by Richard Oden
Cancer statistics reprinted with permission from the American Cancer Society's
"1977 Facts and Figures"

Clinical consultants
Jeanne Rogers, RN, MEd, *Associate Director of Nursing, American
Oncologic Hospital-Fox Chase Cancer Center, Philadelphia.*
Joanne Tully, RN, MPH, *Senior Nurse Coordinator, Delaware Cancer
Network, Wilmington.*
Lillian R. Gigliotti, RN, MSN, *Director of Oncology Nursing and Assistant
Clinical Professor of Nursing, University of Pennsylvania Hospitals,
Philadelphia.*

Library of Congress catalog card number 77-85315
ISBN 0-916730-06-9

CONTENTS

AUTHORS

Alyson J. Bochow is a clinical research nurse in the surgery/oncology clinic at the UCLA Medical Center, Los Angeles. She graduated from the Grace-New Haven School of Nursing, Yale-New Haven Medical Center, Conn.

Nancy Burns is assistant instructor at the University of Texas at Arlington School of Nursing. She received her BS from Texas Christian University and her MS from Texas Woman's University.

Priscilla Butts is a clinical supervisor in gynecology at Thomas Jefferson University Hospital, Philadelphia. She received her BSN from Dillard University, New Orleans, and her MSN from the University of Pennsylvania.

Susan Golden Desotell, currently a private duty nurse in Los Angeles, was formerly head nurse at Sidney Farber Cancer Center in Boston. She has served as associate coordinator for the Gastro-Intestinal Tumor Study Group sponsored by the National Cancer Institute.

Carolyn St. John Elliott, currently a MSN student, was formerly a radiation oncology nurse at the University of Chicago Hospitals and Clinics and at Rhode Island Hospital in Providence.

Patricia Gault, a medical/surgical nurse at Mt. Sinai Hospital in Minneapolis, has developed numerous urology teaching pamphlets. She earned her BSN and MEd degrees from the University of Minnesota.

Sandra Herrman is permanent team leader of a medical oncology unit at American Oncologic Hospital-Fox Chase Cancer Center, Philadelphia. She graduated from Bucks County Community College, Newtown, Pa.

Jacqueline Lamanske is head nurse and enterostomal therapist in the colon and rectal surgery department of Carle Clinic, Urbana, Ill. She graduated from St. Joseph's School of Nursing in Alton, Ill.

Rebecca Malik is an instructor at the senior level at Bryn Mawr Hospital School of Nursing in Bryn Mawr, Pa.

Lisa Begg Marino is director of the University of Pittsburgh Office of Oncology and Regional Cancer Center of Western Pennsylvania. She also founded the Oncology Nursing Society, an educationally oriented organization for oncology nurse specialists.

Edwina A. McConnell is assistant director of surgical nursing at Madison General Hospital in Madison, Wisc. She holds a BS from Boston University and a MS from the University of Colorado.

Pamela S. Peters is nurse coordinator of Cancer Control Activities at American Oncologic Hospital-Fox Chase Cancer Center, Philadelphia. She graduated from Widener College.

Jeanne Rogers is associate director of nursing at American Oncologic Hospital-Fox Chase Cancer Center, Philadelphia. She received her master's degree from Temple University.

Laura Terrill is director of nursing education and former clinical specialist for Wilmington Medical Center, Del. She received her master's degree from the University of Pennsylvania.

Joanne Tully is senior nurse coordinator for the Delaware Cancer Network. She received her bachelor's degree from Villanova University and her master's from the University of Pennsylvania and the University of North Carolina.

Margaret Van Meter is clinical director for *Nursing77* magazine. She formerly was associated with Hahnemann Medical College and Hospital, Philadelphia, where for many years she was head nurse of the cardiothoracic surgical unit.

Beatrice Wagner is assistant professor of medical/surgical nursing at the University of Delaware, Wilmington. She is a clinical nurse specialist in long-term care.

FOREWORD

Caring for cancer patients is as old as the disease itself — and as new as the many roles in which today's nurse is involved. To some people, the words cancer nursing conjure up the image of tumor wards, a hush-hush attitude, and fear of telling a patient his disease, treatment, and prognosis. Nothing could be further from reality. Public information has helped to allay the fear and stigma of cancer. And physicians, nurses, and other health professionals are working together as a team to prevent and detect the disease, as well as cure and rehabilitate patients. In fact, we now cure quite a few patients who have cancer; and some of the remaining ones can expect control of their disease for a number of years.

Whether you realize it or not, you're a vital part of this battle against cancer. You may be involved as a generalist, specialist, practitioner, independent practitioner, educator, or researcher. Your sphere of practice may range from a comprehensive cancer center to a community outreach program, from a general hospital to a physician's office. Wherever you practice, your responsibility encompasses prevention, detection, and rehabilitation. But if you're like most nurses, you contribute most during the curative, rehabilitative, and terminal phases of the disease.

Surgery is the oldest form of treatment for cancer. But advances are still being made in it...and even greater advances are being made in radiation, chemotherapy, and immunotherapy. Whichever treatment or combination of treatments is used, you may be involved in it: administering chemotherapy and treating its side effects; preventing a hemorrhage in a patient after a prostatectomy; or teaching a patient with a laryngectomy how to suction his laryngectomy tube and maintain an open airway.

Undoubtedly, you'll also be involved in giving psychological support. Cancer's psychological impact on patients and their families can be devastating, but frequently you'll see evidence of inner strengths and resources in their courage and active participation in treatment and rehabilitation. You can help them build on their strength. Be sensitive to the patient's psychosocial, as well as his physical needs: See him as a whole person, who has a disease — cancer. You can help the patient and his family adjust to whatever changes occur in their lives because of his treatment, and aid him in planning realistic short- and long-term goals consistent with his life-style and disease.

Do you have the proper armamentarium — the updated skills and sensitivity necessary for the job? This Skillbook will give you that competency, as well as help you define your role in caring for cancer patients. It doesn't dwell on the special problems of terminal patients, which are presented with great sensitivity in the *Nursing Skillbook* DEALING WITH DEATH AND DYING. Instead it focuses on what you can do to help patients who still are fighting for their lives. It discusses the most common cancers, how they are currently treated, and the specific nursing care required for each. The Skillchecks at the end of each section provide you with an opportunity not found in most other cancer nursing books — a chance to test your skills and assess your competence.

Working with cancer patients is one of the most exciting and rewarding ways you can continue your practice. You'll find it rich in opportunities to be innovative, assist other health professionals, and expand your role. Moreover, you'll gain that personal satisfaction you get when you use your professional expertise to help your patient and his family.

RENILDA HILKEMEYER, RN, BS
Assistant to the President
The University of Texas System – Cancer Center
M.D. Anderson Hospital and Tumor Institute
Houston, Texas

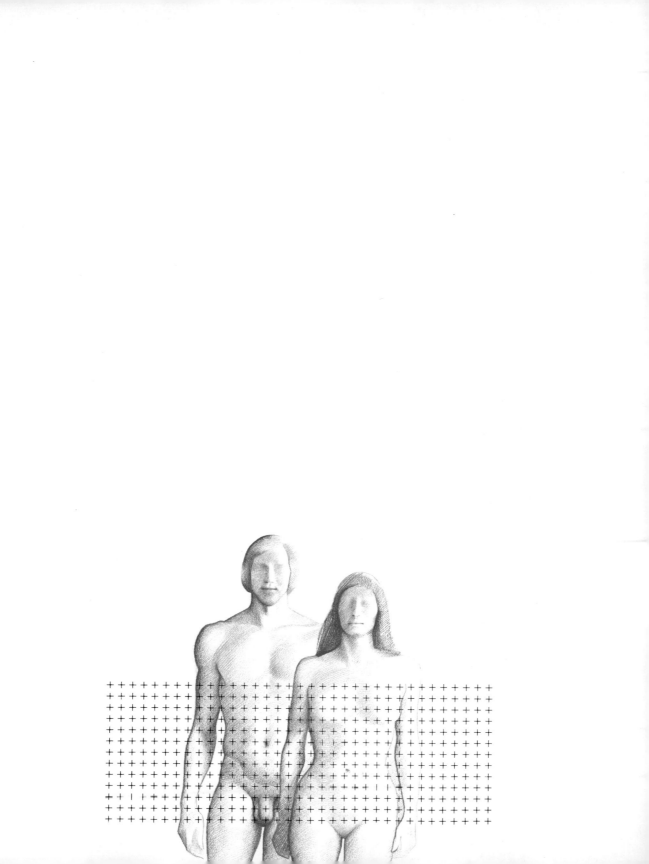

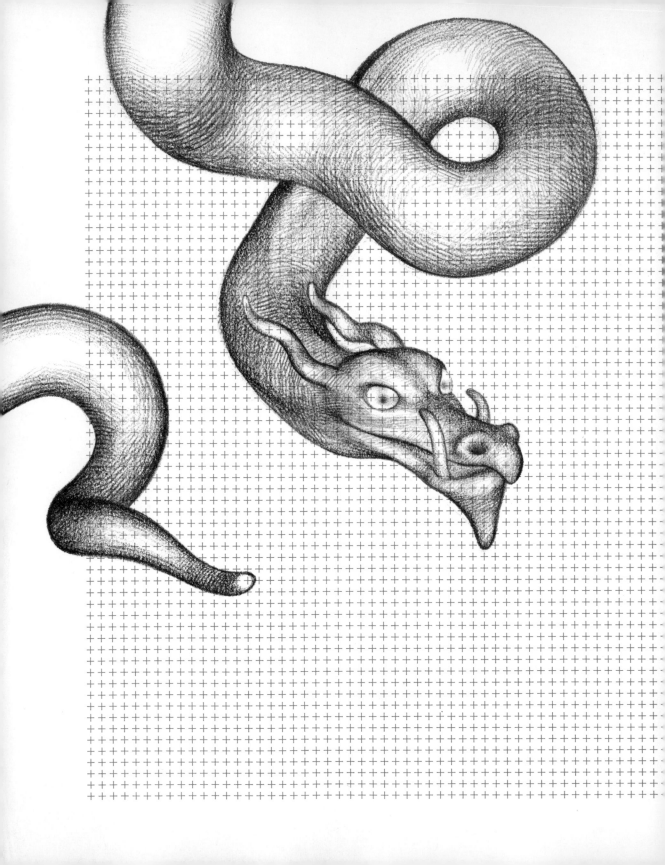

PUTTING YOUR TASK
INTO PERSPECTIVE

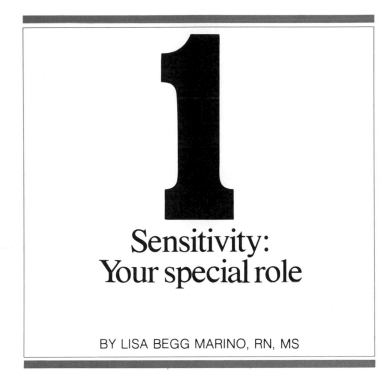

Sensitivity:
Your special role

BY LISA BEGG MARINO, RN, MS

WHY ARE THE WORDS "terminal" and "incurable" most often linked with cancer? Old age is incurable, and there's nothing more terminal than a head-on collision at 70 m.p.h. And every day more people die of heart disease than of cancer.

Though it may be unrealistic and illogical, the fact is that most people (including most health professionals) view cancer with a special dread. And this dread can affect our care of cancer patients. For some of you, a patient who has cancer is depressing and you're reluctant to commit yourself fully to him. If that's the case, maybe it's because in your own mind you're separating cancer patients from other patients, putting them into a special category. Maybe you still haven't emotionally accepted the fact that cancer is just one more chronic disease that needs continuous or periodic treatment.

I know how you're feeling because working with cancer patients depressed me too at first. I was not always a "cancer nurse," or at least I didn't think so. However, in reality, I was a cancer nurse because so many of my patients had cancer. I did not work in some exotic research unit; I worked in a major surgery unit of a general hospital. Most patients I cared for had cancer of some sort. Many had problems secondary to cancer

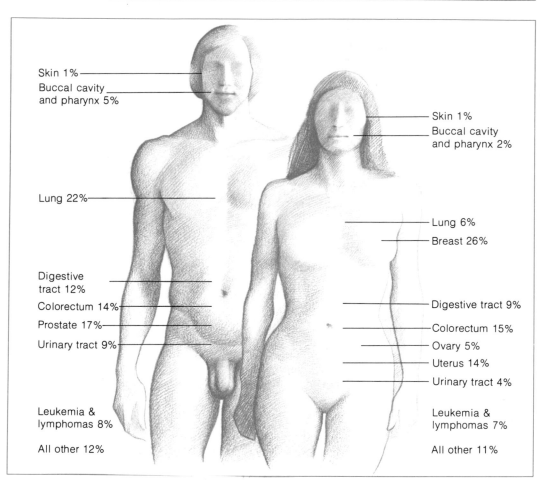

Skin 1%
Buccal cavity and pharynx 5%
Lung 22%
Digestive tract 12%
Colorectum 14%
Prostate 17%
Urinary tract 9%
Leukemia & lymphomas 8%
All other 12%

Skin 1%
Buccal cavity and pharynx 2%
Lung 6%
Breast 26%
Digestive tract 9%
Colorectum 15%
Ovary 5%
Uterus 14%
Urinary tract 4%
Leukemia & lymphomas 7%
All other 11%

Who gets it?
Cancer is the second leading cause of death in the United States and Canada. In 1977 alone, approximately 690,000 new cases were diagnosed in the United States representing a rate of one out of four individuals. The figures above provide a breakdown by site and sex. They do not include non-melanoma skin cancer and carcinoma of the uterine cervix, which are almost 100% curable.

such as obstruction and fistulas. I became overwhelmed by the dimensions of care they required.

Gradually though, I began to realize that I had to redefine my ideas of "success" and "failure." I had equated success with curing people. But the best that medicine has to offer a large percentage of patients is remission. It enables people to live with their disease — much as diabetics do. And, as with diabetics, success in nursing care of cancer can be defined as promoting optimum adaptation to the disease.

I also read that cancer is a very stressful and isolating disease — not only for cancer patients but also for those who care for cancer patients. I realized my experience of emotional exhaustion was by no means unique; others react similarly to suffering. This realization helped me identify a serious problem: I had no one to help me recover my emotional losses.

Fortunately, I was able to talk out my problems with a psychiatric nurse, who explained what was happening to me. "You are grieving because so many of your patients are seriously ill or dying," she said. "Go where there's laughter and joy, and bring some of that joy into your patients' lives."

I also reexamined my attitude toward caring for these patients. My whole attitude was negative because I had only negative experiences: anxious patients and their families awaiting diagnosis, those patients recovering from major surgery, and those admitted with a new crisis. Thanks to our treatment, patients did experience happy interludes between hospitalizations, but we saw only the hospitalizations. Seeing or hearing from a patient during his better times can help you tremendously to preserve your perspective.

You can talk to the community health nurse about your patient, or visit him during an outpatient appointment, or have him visit you. Ask your patient to call you to say hello — he'll do it. He also needs to know that you're interested in his whole life, not just the bad parts. And if you know that there *are* good times, it will help balance out the negative, stressful times.

To tell or not to tell
The next problem I tackled was the age-old question "to tell or not to tell." The fact that it remains a problem only reinforces the fact that many people are still unable to deal openly with cancer — and that goes for many physicians. Unfortunately, this can paralyze a nurse — from fear of being forced to disclose the diagnosis, and from frustration and anger toward the physician or the patient's family.

The nurse, however, has an alternative: to bring all these people together. For example, take a physician who refuses to disclose the diagnosis. As a nurse, you can be a fact finder. By a patient's probing questions, you can assess his level of understanding and his capacity to be told. You can usually validate your observations by merely allowing the patient to talk and share with you his fears and feelings. Then, organize your observations and facts, and approach the physician. But make that approach as one professional to another and be tactful. Many times a physician doesn't tell because he can't. He may have the same fears you do. Make your recommenda-

Beat the odds:
Five-year survival
rates
This chart shows
5-year survival rates for
cancer in selected
sites, comparing
regional and localized
involvement. Although
individual cases vary,
most patients with a
history of cancer are
considered cured if no
evidence of the disease
reappears in five years
after diagnosis. As you
can see, a patient's
chances for survival
greatly increase if his
cancer can be treated
while it is still localized.
In fact, experts estimate
that, with early
detection, half of all
cancer patients could
be saved.

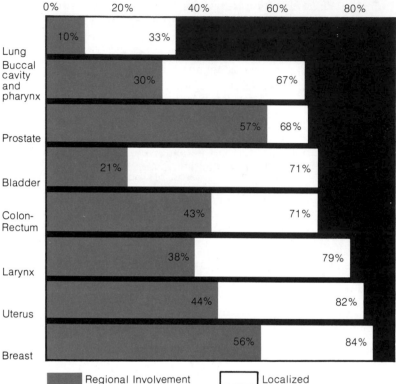

Regional Involvement   Localized

*Adjusted for normal life expectancy.

tion and indicate that you wish to go with him when he tells the
patient.

The other aspect, the family's refusal to permit disclosure,
can be just as destructive because it does not allow the patient
to utilize his major support group. Families who deny the
reality become more like spectators than participants in a
loving relationship.

Here again, if resourceful, you can bridge the gap. You can
talk with the patient, assess his perspective and communicate
this to the family. Usually, the patient already suspects something because of changing interactions, and the family feels
guilty about holding back the truth. Someone has to bring them
together — and that someone can be you. This can be one of
the most satisfying rewards in cancer nursing.

Care, not cure
Now we are at the point of actually caring for the patient with

cancer. Again, the positive approach can work. You don't have to regard your patients as curable or incurable; instead, focus on promoting control of the disease. Control is a much more useful term, for it reflects the chronicity of cancer. More and more our knowledge of cancer rehabilitation is permitting us to assist the patient more effectively. Even if your support comes at the end of a patient's life, it matters a great deal.

Cancer tends to be a prolonged battle, one that may have acute crises and successive, but sometimes temporary, remissions. It may require many alterations in life-style and function. Focusing on the patient's adaptation to his maximum level of functioning can permit you the flexibility to reassess, readjust, readvise, but still remain a supportive care provider. You are not under the pressure to cure, as a physician is. If you *care* and comfort, you are successful.

Set your measure of achievement by what each of your patients can do, considering his special situation. Help him to live life as normally as possible. For instance, the patient who is under treatment for recurrent cancer may still feel well enough to work. If you are the nurse seeing him for follow-up visits, schedule him at 7:30 in the morning, or after 5:00 in the evening, or on a Saturday morning. This will assist him to continue to do something he values while still receiving his treatment.

Every patient has individual needs. One of my patients, who required weekly treatment for metastatic cancer, wanted to take his son on a camping trip. He knew that he could not afford to miss his treatments and asked us for help in solving this problem. We determined the location of his trip and the nearest hospital to it. We then arranged for him to receive treatment at that hospital on a weekly basis for the 3 weeks he was on vacation. In other words, we helped him live a near-normal life.

We are all living
This leads into my last discovery of positive approaches: to do away with the negative "death and dying" attitude. Too often we nurses fall into the pattern of thinking of cancer patients as dying people. We need to remember, instead, that they are also in the process of living. Right now, they are living first — and dying second — as we all are. Our job is to help make that living process as meaningful to them as possible.

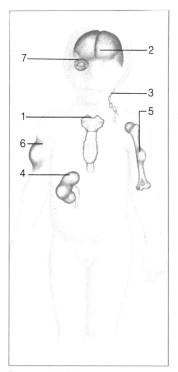

Cancer in kids
Cancer kills more children between the ages of 3 to 14 than any other disease. Acute lymphocytic leukemia causes approximately half of the childhood deaths due to cancer. The figure above shows the seven most common sites of juvenile cancer in order of frequency: 1) hemopoietic sites, indicated by the manubrium; 2) brain and central nervous system; 3) lymphatic system; 4) kidney; 5) bone; 6) connective tissues; and 7) eye and orbit.

By focusing on living, you give your patient and family the benefit of your resourcefulness and coordinating skills. Cancer patients sometimes require baby-sitters, housekeepers, supplies and equipment, nutritional hints when appetites are low; in short, ideas for continuing to live as normally as possible when they are compromised.

If a cancer patient prefers home treatment to hospitalization, it can often be managed if you give your support to those concerned to try such a venture.

Sometimes the experience is surprisingly rewarding. I remember a former patient, a top executive, who was diagnosed as having cancer of the thyroid. In discussing the situation with him and his wife, I soon discovered that they resented each other — she because he shut her out of his life, and he because she couldn't do anything right. He knew that he was going to require constant care and wanted to be in the hospital where "it would be done properly."

In talking alone to the wife, I found out that she really wanted to take care of her husband at home. "I want to feel needed by him just once in my life," she said. We gave her detailed instructions as to his care, finally persuaded the husband to give it a try, and sent them both home. A month later, when they returned for a follow-up visit, the change in them was remarkable. She had proved beyond question that he needed her greatly, and he was impressed and touched by her warm and efficient care. Although he survived only another year, it was a year in which they were closer to each other than ever before.

These are just some of the crucial problems facing nurses who work with cancer patients. The important information to consider is that the cancer situation is improving. Many more patients are surviving, and still others are surviving with some residual cancer. They need someone who can help them adjust and live, perhaps with limitations, but still able to carry on with things they value. You can do much to facilitate this adaptation, but only if you are able to view your cancer patient not as a dying person, but as a living challenge.

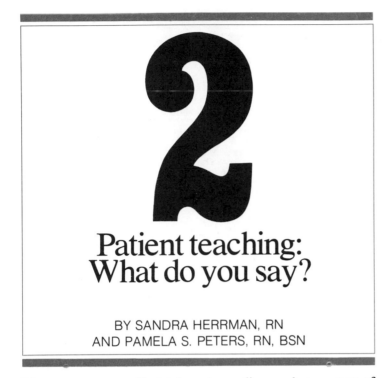

Patient teaching:
What do you say?

BY SANDRA HERRMAN, RN
AND PAMELA S. PETERS, RN, BSN

WHAT IS CANCER? Certainly not one disease, but a group of over 100 different diseases marked by uncontrolled and disordered growth of abnormal cells. If any of these diseases goes unchecked, it will eventually cause death. In fact, some cancers are so deadly that even health professionals regard them negatively.

What's your responsibility in understanding the nature of cancer? It's considerable if you're to provide good nursing care for your cancer patients. And though the terms used in this chapter may seem very simple to you, they're that way for a reason — to explain the disease to your patients. If they ask, you can tell them how cancer cells behave differently from normal cells; how fast and how far they spread when left unchecked; and why they kill.

Wild or self-disciplined
For starters, consider the structure and function of normal cells. They differ widely in appearance and function, because of their location in the body, but they do have much in common. Their reproduction is very precise, orderly, and well controlled. However, the motility of normal cells is limited.

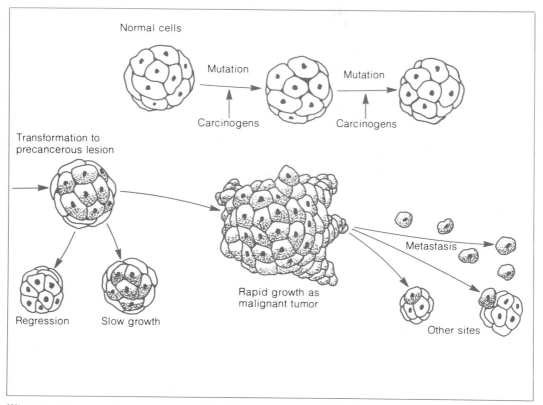

Normal cells

Mutation

Carcinogens

Mutation

Carcinogens

Transformation to
precancerous lesion

Regression

Slow growth

Rapid growth as
malignant tumor

Metastasis

Other sites

What causes cancer?

The cause of cancer remains unknown. One theory of how it begins goes like this: Carcinogens in the environment — X-rays, radioactive elements, organic chemicals (such as benzidine, tobacco products, and coal tar), and inorganic agents (such as nickel, asbestos, and arsenic) — induce mutations in a single line of cells. At some point, the cells may transform into a precancerous lesion that may either regress, develop slowly, or grow rapidly into a malignant tumor. Cancerous cells may then break off from the primary site, metastasizing through the blood or lymphatic system to establish tumors in other parts of the body.

What keeps normal cells from moving about indiscriminately? Two things: adhesion (the tendency of like cells to stick together) and contact inhibition of motion (the cessation of movement when one cell adheres to another).

Malignant cells, on the other hand, are characterized in part by uncontrolled motility. They also have two other common characteristics that distinguish them from normal cells: uncontrolled functioning and uncontrolled division.

As cells become malignant, they lose their specialized structure and function within an organism. This makes more of them reproduce and divide at a greater rate than normal cells. Malignant cells are less adhesive and tend to dissociate more easily from their original location. They don't form regular layers, as normal cells do even in culture, but move about and pile in a disordered, random fashion.

This lack of adhesion and loss of contact inhibition permits cancer to metastasize — leave its primary site and start growing in another part of the body.

ESSENTIAL DIFFERENCES BETWEEN BENIGN AND MALIGNANT TUMORS		
CHARACTERISTIC	BENIGN	MALIGNANT
Growth	Slow expansion; push aside surrounding tissue but do not infiltrate.	Rapid infiltration of surrounding tissues, extending in all directions.
Limitation	Frequently encapsulated.	Seldom encapsulated; ill-defined.
Recurrence	When removed surgically, do not recur	When removed surgically, frequently recur due to infiltration into surrounding tissues
Morphology	Cells closely resemble those of tissue of origin	Cells vary abnormally from those of tissue of origin
Differentiation	Great differentiation	Poor or no differentiation
Mitotic activity	Slight	Usually great
Tissue destruction	Minimal	Extensive due to infiltration and metastatic lesion
Spread	Do not spread; remain localized	Spread via blood and/or lymph systems; establish secondary tumors
Effect on body	No cachexia. Usually do not kill but may obstruct vital organs, exert pressure, produce excess hormones. Can become malignant	Typical cachexia — anemia, loss of weight, weakness, etc. Always kill if not removed surgically or treated promptly before metastasis

Is it benign or deadly?

When any group of cells behaves abnormally, it can form a benign or malignant neoplasm in any part of the body capable of cell division. (See table above for a comparison between neoplasms.)

Neoplasms differ widely in appearance and behavior; there are benign, hyperplastic tumors that regress; benign tumors that remain localized; dependent tumors that grow only if certain hormonal or other conditions are met; tumors that metastasize; and rapidly aggressive tumors.

Pathologists classify malignant neoplasms by parent tissue. Carcinomas start in epithelial tissues (those covering external and internal body surfaces, such as skin, lung and gastrointestinal linings). Sarcomas arise from nonepithelial tissues, such as bone, muscle, fat, cartilage, lymphoid, or hematopoietic cells.

A tumor's original location and cell class determine its name. For example, a malignancy of epithelial basal cells is a

basal cell carcinoma; a malignancy of bone cells is an os-
teogenic sarcoma.

Not all tumors are malignant, of course. However, some
benign tumors later become malignant. Why this happens is
not clearly understood, but scientists have several theories.
Sometimes chronic exposure to carcinogenic agents causes
the transformation — though many precancerous tumors remain benign throughout exposure. Still others become malignant with no exposure. This paradox has convinced some
scientists that factors within a person's body play a part in
origination of malignancy.

To survive and grow, a malignant tumor needs oxygen,
nutrients, and an adequate blood supply from its host. So it
enlarges the blood vessels around itself and forms new ones,
increasing the blood supply to and within tumor. Sometimes,
though, a cancer grows too large and too fast to get the nutrients it needs, so necrosis develops, causing ulceration and
bleeding.

How cancers spread

A malignant tumor metastasizes by invading the surrounding
normal tissue, penetrating blood and lymph vessels and starting secondary tumors in other sites. A rapidly growing tumor
often creates local pressure by squeezing tumor cells into
areas along paths of least resistance. First, it invades soft
tissue, then it crosses into veins and lymph vessels. Lastly, it
infiltrates the most resistant tissue — organ capsules, cartilage, arterial walls, and dense, fibrous areas.

When malignant cells enter blood and lymph vessels, they
metastasize, traveling to distant body sites and starting new
tumors. Not every cell survives the trip, however. Some get
destroyed by agitation, mechanical injury during passage, or
by the host's immunological defenses.

Despite the lymph nodes' role as defenders against disease,
they are apt to capture cancer cells and let them grow, especially when the primary tumor is a carcinoma. This secondary
cell group then may invade neighboring nodes. And where
lymph nodes drain into subclavian veins, the cells can go
further, entering the bloodstream.

However, bloodstream metastasis is less predictable than
lymph system metastasis. Cancerous emboli are sometimes
trapped in small or irregular capillaries. When cancer cells do

get through the bloodstream, though, they are more likely to invade highly vascular organs. Before a cancerous embolism can metastasize, it must reach receptive tissue.

Tumor vs. host

A malignant tumor is like a parasite; it needs a host — or, in this case, a body — to survive and grow. Although a malignant tumor depends on its host in this way, it frequently winds up killing the host and itself. The relationship between malignant tumor and host is usually one-sided in the tumor's favor, though the host's reaction — and the medical treatment given — influence the outcome.

A malignant tumor's attack on its host is many leveled, in the cells, tissues, bloodstream, and lymphatic system. How severely the host is affected by this attack depends on the tumor's location, its growth, and the stage of the disease. Generally, cancer's effect on the host increases as the disease progresses.

Because an early tumor is frequently localized, the first problems it causes for the host are relatively small. Damage to surrounding normal cells (and their subsequent death) usually occurs first. This happens when the tumor invades and compresses local tissues, decreasing the protective fluid that cells need to survive, and shutting off their blood supply. Necrosis results.

Tumor pressure may also produce a variety of other symptoms — mild numbness, tingling, and pain from pressure on nerve fibers. Local edema occurs when normal passage of lymph fluid is blocked. When pressure blocks the urinary or gastrointestinal systems, it can threaten life.

As the tumor grows, so do the number and severity of problems. Tissue necrosis ultimately leads to adverse systemic disorders — or superimposed complications. For example, an ulcerated tumor breaking through the skin or organ mucosa may start a secondary infection. Or it may cause a severe hemorrhage, due to its highly vascular nature. Steadily increasing pain also develops.

When the cancer becomes far advanced, all these problems cause cachexia — a state of profound ill health and malnutrition. As the host wastes, the tumor continues to grow, producing more debilitating symptoms. Eventually, death comes — killing both host and tumor.

Pain: A fate worse than death?
Some patients fear the pain of cancer as much as or more than death. But generally pain occurs only in the advanced stages — most commonly in cancer of the cervix, lungs, rectum, and prostate.

The severity of pain will vary from patient to patient. But you can generally identify the severity by certain signs and symptoms. Tachycardia, for instance, usually indicates superficial pain; bradycardia, on the other hand, indicates severe, deep pain. Nausea, vomiting, and rapid, shallow breathing are also hallmarks of severe pain.

Although you can't assure a patient that he won't have pain, you can assure him that you'll do everything possible to relieve it.

• *Simple nursing measures.* Back rubs, changing position, and just listening can take the edge off minor pain.

• *Medications.* For early, minor pain, the doctor may order mild medications such as aspirin (10 gr) or aspirin combined with propoxyphene (Darvon, 32-65 mg) or codeine (15-30 mg). For severe pain, he may order tranquilizers or narcotics such as merperidine (Demerol, 50-100 mg), pantopium (Pantopon, 5-20 mg), or hydromorphone (Dilaudid, 2-4 mg).

• *Radiation.* This can ease the pains of metastasis, particularly to the bones and brain.

• *Surgery.* Doctors usually reserve surgery for excruciating pain in terminal patients. Procedures include nerve blocks, alcohol injections, cordotomy (for pain in the upper thorax only), spinothalamic tractotomy (for the arms, shoulders, and neck), posterior rhizotomy (for the trigeminal, glossopharyngeal, and cervical plexuses), and prefrontal leucotomy (for the patient's *reaction* to pain).

Classifying cancer

Staging varies from site to site within the body, and cancer centers throughout the country use different systems. But one common system is the TNM system: T for primary tumor, N for regular lymph nodes, and M for distant metastasis. The following designations extend the classifications:

TUMOR

TO: No evidence of primary tumor.

TIS: Carcinoma in situ

T1, T2, T3, T4: Progressive increase in tumor, size, and involvement.

TX: Tumor cannot be assessed.

NODES

NO: Regional lymph nodes not demonstrably abnormal.

N1, N2, N3, etc.: Increasing degrees of demonstrable abnormality of regional lymph nodes. (For many primary sites the subscript "a," e.g. N1a, may indicate that metastasis to the node isn't suspected; and the subscript "b," may indicate that metastasis to the node is suspected or proved.)

NX: Regional lymph nodes cannot be assessed clinically.

METASTASIS

MO: No evidence of distant metastasis.

M1, M2, M3: Ascending degrees of distant metastasis, including metastasis to distant lymph nodes.

Host vs. tumor

How a host affects a malignant tumor is less obvious. Some pathologists believe the host responds with its immunological system. In other words, the host fights the tumor with cellular immunity much the same as it fights any infection or injury. Sometimes this natural, inflammatory response temporarily decreases tumor pressure by removing and repairing necrotic tissue, but it doesn't last — because the tumor remains.

Occasionally, large numbers of malignant cells circulate in a host's body without metastasizing. Scientists theorize that cellular immunity may be responsible for this, though not for spontaneous remissions or disappearance of metastases after surgery has eliminated the primary lesion.

Does the host have any other immune response against cancer? Yes, there's strong evidence that humoral immunity is activated when there's a malignancy. Like cellular immunity, this is an acquired immunity with predominant circulating antibodies. To understand how it works, picture malignant cells developing a distinctive, antigenic profile that attracts cancer-fighting antibodies. Scientists have pinpointed these antigens on plasma membranes of most experimental tumors. If they can unlock the secrets of antigen-antibody responses, they may find a way to control cancer (see Chapter 6).

Humoral and cellular immune responses account for most of the host's antitumor activities. However, the host fights back in still another way — counterpressure. Tumors are sometimes held back temporarily by well-supported body structures like bone and fibrous tissue. Unfortunately, necrosis results when the tumor's blood and oxygen supplies are reduced. Ulceration and bleeding occur, negatively affecting the host.

Will science find a cure?

Will scientists ever discover the solution to cancer's secrets? The research methods used today certainly make victory a reasonable expectation. In the meantime, you can use the simple explanation of cancer in this chapter to improve your oncological nursing skills. Help your patient and his family understand the disease — by answering their questions.

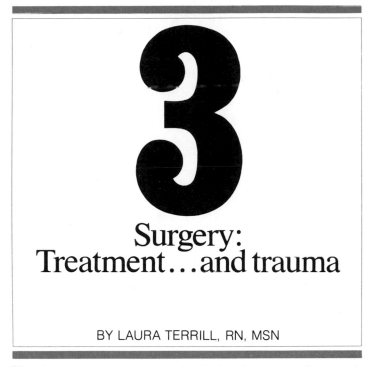

3

Surgery:
Treatment...and trauma

BY LAURA TERRILL, RN, MSN

YOU'RE INTERVIEWING a newly admitted cancer patient who's
scheduled for surgery. As you explain the procedure, you
sense that he isn't listening. How can you get through to him?
Or suppose he accepts the need for surgery but a close member
of the family (on whom he depends for support) says, "I won't
let them do it to you." What then?

If you can't solve problems like these, your physical care of
the patient may not be enough to restore him to health or even
help him cope with his illness. Because radical surgery, particularly if it's mutilating, can create enormous psychological
problems. And these can prevent a patient from participating
in postop care...from learning self-care before discharge...even in extreme cases from going through with life-
saving surgery at all.

In the following chapters you'll learn about particular types
of surgery, the special preop and postop care they demand,
and the particular emotional problems they can create. But
here let's look at the general emotional impact of surgery and
what you can do about it. To help a patient cope, you'll need to
know how to probe his fears, answer touchy questions, and
prepare him for unpleasant aftereffects of surgery.

Getting to know him

Learning that he has cancer — or that he may have cancer — can be devastating enough for a patient. The thought of mutilating surgery, such as a colostomy, can be almost too much for the patient to handle. Even if he may not suffer from any visible mutilation, he may be overwhelmed by the thought of the surgery's effects, such as impotence from prostate surgery. Or he may be less worried about the surgery itself and more worried about his chances for survival, as with lung cancer. In addition to this, he may fear pain, enormous medical costs, losing his job, or losing the love of his family.

Small wonder, then, that a patient may come to you preoccupied, worried, or dazed. To help him cope with his impending surgery, you have to learn his feelings. One of the best ways to do that is through your nursing history interview and follow-up conversation. If the patient has been admitted several days preop in preparation for surgery, you'll have a chance to talk with him several times. This not only lets the patient become comfortable talking about his surgery and gives him time to digest information; it also gives you a good chance to really get to know the patient, to see his moods, and to let him know that you're there when he needs you. You can easily talk while you're making his bed or giving a back rub...anytime when the atmosphere is relaxed. If the patient comes in the day before surgery, you should try to visit him as often as possible.

Recently, in our hospital, we had a patient scheduled for radical removal of her upper palate for adenocystic cancer of the salivary glands. Mrs. K. was 48, the mother of three children, and the wife of a supportive husband. When I interviewed her a week before admission, she seemed remarkably well adjusted to her diagnosis and the impending surgery. Even after she had undergone several days of preop workup, she still seemed quite accepting. I heard the doctor explain that the surgery would cause some facial deformity and that she would need a prosthesis and a skin graft; we made arrangements for an appointment for her at the local maxillofacial unit to get a temporary prosthesis for the upper palate. She seemed to be adjusting to everything.

The day before surgery, I again talked with her about what the surgery would mean — the dietary limitations after surgery, the need for a temporary prosthesis and skin graft, how she would look immediately after surgery. She listened quietly. Then, the night before surgery, as we were discussing final details of the surgery, she finally cried. I think that was her turning point; she was finally moving from denial toward eventual acceptance.

Generally, I find that patients who grieve before surgery, as Mrs. K. did, recover emotionally more quickly than those who enter surgery still seeming to deny their condition. Still, most patients adjust within a few weeks after surgery. If not, they may need psychiatric help.

Before surgery, also introduce the patient to the O.R. personnel and ICU nurses if possible. He'll feel like he at least has some contacts when he is moved from one area to another. And this meeting will help provide continuity of care.

How does the patient expect the surgery to affect him? If the surgery is radical and will change his appearance or limit his activities, will he be devastated? Answers to these questions are tied up with the patient's self-concept and his body image. An attractive young woman scheduled for a mastectomy, for instance, may have far more trouble coping with the idea of surgery than an older woman. The young woman may see her breasts as vital to her sexual attractiveness; an older woman may have less concern about her attractiveness. An aggressive, successful salesman may have more difficulty adjusting to a laryngectomy than a writer. The salesman may consider a strong voice to be essential not only to his job, but also to his identity as a dynamic, persuasive person; a writer, on the other hand, probably wouldn't depend as heavily on his voice for his professional or even personal identity.

I can't give you any firm guidelines on what will be most upsetting to patients; each person is different. But if you ask, "Do you expect this surgery to change your life or your life-style?" most patients will welcome a chance to discuss their concerns.

Of course, you can't deny that the surgery will change a patient's life in some ways. But you can help him come to terms with it by reinforcing the reason for the surgery and the expected benefits (see accompanying list).

If the surgery will be mutilating, the patient may want to discuss the expected deformity. Since the patient may feel more comfortable discussing it with someone who "has been there," you might arrange a visit from a well-adjusted patient

Reasons for surgery

Patients will accept surgery more readily if you can explain to them the reasons behind it.

• *To establish a diagnosis.* Examining a suspicious lesion microscopically (with a biopsy) or visually (with an endoscope or diagnostic laparotomy) confirms or rules out the presence of cancer.

• *To remove a precancerous lesion.* Eliminating benign lesions that have a tendency toward malignant transformation — for example, leukoplakia, colon and rectal polyps, and certain pigmented moles.

• *To stage a disease.* Staging determines the extent of the cancer's invasion, and may be done surgically — as in the staging procedure for Hodgkin's disease.

• *To cure.* An attempt to remove the cancer completely, which, in radical approaches, may necessitate removal of one of the patient's limbs, breasts, organs, or other body parts. When cancer is diagnosed early, surgery may cure the patient without disfigurement.

• *To reconstruct after a radical procedure.* Reconstructive surgery after a mastectomy, radical neck dissection, or other disfiguring procedures may relieve a patient's psychological trauma.

• *To palliate.* When cancer is far advanced and a cure is not probable, surgery may relieve pain, pressure, infection, and hemorrhage. Palliative procedures for intractable pain include: rhizotomy, peripheral neurotomy, cervical or thoracic cordotomy, tractotomy, thalamotomy, sympathectomy, and frontal lobotomy.

Problems with protein
If your patient has a protein deficiency before surgery (as many cancer patients do), it may be due to several things: loss of appetite; chronic loss of blood; malabsorption; inability to swallow; or the nutritional demands of cancer cells. He may need a special diet before surgery to prevent serious difficulties postoperatively: impaired wound healing, upset liver function, reduced resistance to infection, and susceptibility to decubiti.

If the physician decides to delay surgery till the patient's nutritional status is better, he'll probably put the patient on a diet that's high in protein, carbohydrates, and calories — yet low in fat. If the patient can't eat solid foods (or needs a supplement to the above diet), he may receive a liquid dietary formula that's high in protein and calories. This can be a commercial formula or one formulated by the hospital's dietition. Make these supplements more appetizing by freezing them or serving diluted over ice.

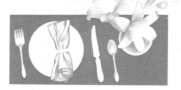

who has recovered from a similar procedure (see Chapters 8 and 9). Not all patients would appreciate a visit though. You have to use your nursing judgment to determine a patient's readiness. Consider the case of Miss S., who was being prepared for a colostomy. Every time we mentioned the stoma before surgery, she became very upset, crying and refusing to talk. Arranging a visit from a rehabilitated ostomy patient at that time probably would've been a mistake. In this particular case, we waited until after surgery. Miss S. refused to look at the stoma for several days. But when she began peeking at it as the nurses changed the appliance, we invited a rehabilitated ostomy patient for a visit. We felt that she needed some encouragement to begin caring for the stoma herself.

How can you make the patient's hospital stay more comfortable? In some cases, the patient may need help from the social service department to arrange transportation to the hospital, financing for his hospitalization, or even babysitting for children at home. If he needs spiritual support, arrange a visit from his hospital chaplain or the patient's own priest, minister, or rabbi.

Often I find that a patient who is hospitalized for tests several days preop becomes anxious about waiting for surgery — particularly if he can only have one test a day. He worries that every day "wasted" means the cancer is more threatening to his life. In such cases, you can only keep explaining the reason for the tests and why they must be scheduled as they are. Between tests, though, you might be able to get the patient a short pass out of the hospital for a trip home, dinner out with a friend or family member — anything to take his mind off his situation, if only briefly. Whether or not you can arrange a pass depends on your hospital's policy and the patient's condition and limitations, of course. If you do arrange one, though, be sure the patient signs a release before leaving, relieving the hospital of all liability while he is away.

Toward the end of your nursing interview, try to get the patient to talk about the cancer and what it means to him. Sometimes you'll find that the conversation just naturally leads in that direction. If not, though, you could ask the patient how he feels about his illness. Or, if he looks worried, say, "You seem worried. What's bothering you?" Nearly all patients will talk freely about their feelings if given this kind of opportunity.

But how can you help a patient overcome his worries? Obviously you can't tell a patient that he won't die, if that's his main concern. That's false assurance — and the patient knows it. But you can emphasize the hopeful side of his condition. the good nurses, skilled doctors, and the advances in cancer treatment available to him. Also tell him about the people you know who had the same disease and recovered.

Sometimes a patient won't directly tell you that he's afraid he'll die. Recently, for example, a woman scheduled for a lobectomy for lung cancer kept saying that she would never see a mountain in Maine that she had always wanted to see. Clearly her real concern was that she was going to die. I couldn't assure her that she would see that mountain, but I told her about another patient who had had a pneumonectomy — and was now recuperating in the Bahamas! That seemed to ease her mind.

Don't assume that all patients are most worried about dying, though. A mother, for instance, might be worried about her husband trying to take care of the children; a businessman might be worried about missing an important meeting; a husband might be worried about his wife's reaction to his illness. You may not be able to actually solve the person's problem. But you can help him realize that, although he can't change the situation, he may have alternatives open to him. The mother, for instance, might be able to ask a friend or babysitter to help with the children one or two nights a week; the businessman could have a colleague represent him at the meeting and call afterwards with a report; the husband could ask a friend or relative to stay with his wife. The important thing is that you help the patient explore the various avenues open to him and get him whatever outside help he may need for an acceptable solution.

Don't forget the family
Don't neglect the family in your preop interview. Since their initial reaction to the patient's appearance after surgery will be so important to his reaction, tell them what tubes, machines, and disfigurement to expect after surgery.

Not all family members can deal with the patient's illness equally well. Try to find one close family member who seems most able to deal with the situation and explain the procedures, as well as the time of surgery and when the patient probably will return to his room. That person then can relay the information to the rest of the family. You might jot down that person's name, address, and phone number in the nursing care plan so you can contact him later in case of emergency.

Try to accept the family's feelings toward the patient; they may range from over-solicitous to resentful. Family values and beliefs may influence your patient's feelings about himself; if so, they will certainly affect his recovery by influencing his cooperation with orders and his participation in rehabilitation activities. If the family needs spiritual support, call the hospital chaplain or encourage a visit from the family's priest, rabbi, or pastor.

Occasionally, a family member has more trouble than the patient coping with impending cancer surgery. We saw such a situation with Mr. P., a 64-year-old, heavy smoker with cancer of the larynx. He was scheduled for a laryngectomy, which he and his wife appeared to accept. But his 24-year-old son tried to prevent it. "No, you can't do that to Dad," he announced defiantly. "I won't let you!" He was so upset by the diagnosis that he was overwhelmed with anger.

To help him overcome his anger, we started by listening and accepting his anger. Then we helped him understand that without the scheduled laryngectomy, his father would die. By agreeing to surgery, however devastating it might be, his father had chosen to live. We assured him that, although his father would live without his normal voice, he could be taught esophageal speech.

The son's anger was dissipated by our acceptance of it and he listened to what we had to say. We then called a member of the Lost Chord Club (American Laryngectomy Association), and with the member's added reassurance, Mr. P.'s son gained strength to support his father's decision. If we hadn't intervened, Mr. P.'s recovery might have been hampered and his full rehabilitation delayed by his distress over his son's negative attitude.

After surgery

What's important postoperatively? Your patient's immediate needs are mainly physical during this crucial time, and include continuous assessment of vital signs, maintenance of a patent airway, prevention of infection and hemorrhage, maintenance of fluid electrolyte balance, and control of pain. Specific nurs-

FIVE-YEAR SURVIVAL RATE FOR SURGERY — MALE

SITE	% TREATED BY SURGERY ALONE*	5-YEAR SURVIVAL RATE	10-YEAR SURVIVAL RATE
Colon	77%	53%	47%
Rectum	72%	59%	41%
Lip	76%	90%	84%
Salivary	82%	90%	86%
Floor of mouth	37%	54%	39%
Other mouth	33%	66%	56%
Thyroid	54%	89%	87%
Bladder	73%	69%	61%
Kidney	52%	56%	44%
Larynx	43%	68%	61%
Prostate	36%***	55%	34%
Stomach	43%	23%	19%

FIVE-YEAR SURVIVAL RATE FOR SURGERY — FEMALE

SITE	% TREATED BY SURGERY ALONE*	5-YEAR SURVIVAL RATE	10-YEAR SURVIVAL RATE
Breast	57%	75%	62%
Colon	77%	58%	52%
Rectum	72%	52%	46%
Lip	76%	94%	82%**
Salivary	88%	97%	96%
Floor of mouth	47%	64%	58%**
Other mouth	44%	75%	68%
Thyroid	66%	95%	94%
Uterus	23%	84%	81%
Ovary	23%	54%	48%
Bladder	71%	71%	65%
Kidney	56%	54%	46%
Larynx	37%	69%	57%**
Stomach	42%	28%	24%

All rates age-adjusted.
* Figures based on reporting tumor registries only, 1955-1964
** Includes between 5%-10% margin of error
*** Prostate statistics based on treatment with surgery, chemotherapy, and hormones

Courtesy: National Cancer Institute End Results Study Group, 1972

ing care for the most common cancer surgery procedures are outlined throughout this book.

After surgery, reinforce what you've taught your patient and his family preoperatively. They may have been too upset to understand everything before, or perhaps they just wouldn't listen. Prepare the family once again for any tubes or machines the patient will have, as well as any physical alterations, so they won't upset him by reacting unfavorably. If the surgery was extensive or disfiguring, expect the patient to have some adjustment difficulties.

Don't ever discourage the patient from talking about his surgery or disease; it may be his way of testing you to see if he's still acceptable. If he says something like "How can you stand looking at me?" or "I must be disgusting," try turning the question around. Say, "What is there about it that seems so unpleasant to you?" This turns the conversation away from *your* feelings, toward *his* feelings. If your attitude stays reassuring and positive, the patient will gain strength to adapt to his body changes.

Occasionally, you'll have a patient who refuses to look at his surgical site and wants no part of the self-care that goes with rehabilitation. Mr. B., who'd undergone a colostomy, was this kind of patient. He called himself a freak and didn't want his wife to visit him. He refused to watch or participate in stoma care.

We tried to discover what bothered him most. Was it fear of rejection? Or loss of body function control? In Mr. B.'s case, it was a little bit of both. We introduced him to some rehabilitated teachers and businessmen from the United Ostomy Association. When he quit referring to himself as a freak, we realized that he had finally adjusted.

Toward rehabilitation and self-care
You can help make your patient's life worth living again by utilizing all the social, financial, and vocational resources at your disposal...by focusing on his total needs...by reinforcing a positive self-image. But keep in mind that surgery may have been just part of his total treatment plan. So you may have to prepare him for what comes next — perhaps radiation treatments, or chemotherapy.

4

Radiation:
A focused assault

BY CAROLYN ST. JOHN ELLIOTT, RN, BS

BECAUSE CANCER PATIENTS have a chronic disease, they need continuous treatment. Gone are the days when a surgeon operated on a cancer patient and sent him home with the hope that surgery had done the job. Today, treatment is inevitably multimodal, with palliation or permanent or temporary remission the goals. Radiation is one such treatment modality — and new techniques have greatly improved its effectiveness.

Unfortunately, though, radiation oncology has been misunderstood by many patients — and some nurses as well.

Since about one half of all cancer patients receive radiation therapy at some time during their overall treatment, you should be aware of how radiation affects them.

Myths have arisen about this therapy, perhaps because the patient is treated by huge machines located off the beaten track of the hospital. The fact that the patient is subjected to strange rays, alone in a windowless room, has seemed dehumanizing and has been hard to accept by some. And sometimes the disadvantages of radiation therapy seem to override the advantages of treatment.

Even before treatment, you can be one of the main supports to the patient. You may be the one who has to answer the

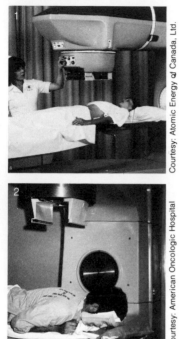

Courtesy: Atomic Energy of Canada, Ltd.

Courtesy: American Oncologic Hospital

Getting below the surface
Two machines basic to radiotherapy today are the cobalt$_{60}$ unit (figure 1), and the linear accelerator (figure 2). They can deliver a high amount of radiation to the tumor without being limited by the tissue tolerance of the skin. At 2 megavolts (MeV), the cobalt$_{60}$ delivers 50% of the dose to 10 cm below the skin level. The linear accelerator produces between 6 and 35 MeV and delivers up to 90% of its dose to a depth of 10 cm.

At these high energies the edges of the beam are very sharp, with little side-scatter. The higher the energy, the better the quality of the beam produced. The better the quality of the beam, the more precisely the therapist can deliver a cancercidal dose to the tumor without damage to the surrounding tissue and bone.

patient's questions about the upcoming treatment. You may have to explain what the patient will go through and the possible side effects. But only if you understand fully the treatment of cancer by radiation therapy can you help your patient face the unknown.

That is what we tried to do with Mrs. F., who came to our gynecology-oncology clinic for radiation treatment on an outpatient basis. She had carcinoma of the ovary, Stage IIA, and 4 weeks earlier she had had a hysterectomy and a bilateral salpingo-oophorectomy. When she first came to us, she was apprehensive and full of questions. We answered them one by one.

What is radiation treatment? The radiation therapist can use two modes of treatment: external and internal. With external radiation, a machine, usually some distance from the patient, delivers X-rays or gamma rays to a lesion on or in the patient's body. With internal radiation an isotope is placed intracavitarily or interstitially with the same therapeutic effect. Mrs. F.'s treatment would be external.

What does the treatment accomplish? Radiation therapy is not a last-ditch effort to salvage a patient. In our department 50 percent of our patients are treated to cure. The rest can look forward to improvement of the quality of their lives.

The radiation treatment of cancer falls into three categories: curative (primary treatment), palliative, or as an adjunct to other therapies. For example, radiation therapy, the treatment of choice with Stage I or II Hodgkin's disease, is curative in many cases. Radiation therapy for breast cancer is palliative; it may not extend the patient's life, but it does reduce pain from bone mestastases or drainage from chest wall mestastases. Finally, radiation therapy is an adjunct to chemotherapy or surgery when they are the treatments of choice. Such was the case with Mrs. F.

Will radiation damage other parts of the body? The radiation oncologist tries to deliver a maximal dose to the tumor and a minimal dose to the surrounding normal tissue. He does not always succeed and normal cells may be damaged. Much of this damage is acute, lasting until the end of treatment or shortly afterwards. Internal organs sensitive to radiation are most affected and must be protected. In a patient like Mrs. F., who would receive abdominal radiation, 100 percent kidney blocks would be made to shield her kidneys.

What side effects will radiation cause? Most of the time, serious complications do not occur. However, since radiation often causes temporary cell damage — particularly in the gastrourinary tract — Mrs. F., and patients with similar radiation treatments, may experience extreme fatigue, anorexia, vomiting, diarrhea, and urinary frequency. Some skin damage and a drop in blood count might also occur.

Mrs. F. started her treatment with whole abdomen irradiation trimmed down to a banjo at 3000 rads (banjo-port including the entire pelvis with extension up to include the periaortic lymph nodes). This port was reduced again at 5000 rads to give an additional 1000 rads just to the pelvic port, bringing the total dose to the area of the primary to 6000 rads.

At the same time we instituted measures to help lessen the expected side effects. We placed her on a special diet and encouraged her to develop good eating habits, emphasizing the necessity of maintaining her weight to speed tissue repair. But to do that, she had to be on a diet that she liked and one that would also help prevent nausea and diarrhea. We put her on a high-protein, high-carbohydrate, fat-free, low-residue diet to reduce bulk and maintain calories.

Side effects — as expected

Despite our precautions, Mrs. F. developed severe nausea. We gave her prochlorperazine (Compazine, Stemetil) and advised her as follows: Don't eat for several hours before treatment; don't be in the same room where food is prepared; eat several small meals instead of three large ones; eat with the family (family meals are associated with companionship, and tend to stimulate appetite) and drink plenty of fluids, to help replace the fluid loss incurred through vomiting and diarrhea.

Mrs. F. followed the diet but still developed severe diarrhea. The therapist reduced her abdominal field after 2000 rads, and we gave her diphenoxylate hydrochloride (Lomotil). Both would help alleviate the diarrhea. We also gave her a low-residue, easily absorbed diet supplement, which helped maintain fluid intake and increased nutritional intake.

Mrs. F. never developed hematuria or urinary frequency, which are usually acute side effects of bladder irradiation. Her blood count did drop, and she was given transfusions and rest from treatment.

Every patient who receives radiation therapy runs the risk

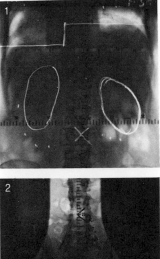

Block that ray
To minimize the destruction of healthy tissues, each radiation patient has individually fashioned shields. Post IVP (Figure1) shows the position of Mrs. F.'s kidneys in relation to the top of the port (line at top) so a shield can be designed to protect them. Figure 2 shows a banjo port encompassing the para-aortic lymph nodes (shown with dye in them) and almost the entire bony pelvis.

AMERICAN CANCER SOCIETY SAMPLE DIET
FOR PATIENTS UNDERGOING RADIATION THERAPY

BREAKFAST	SERVING PORTION	SAMPLE MENU
Fruit	½ cup	Orange juice
Cereal	½ cup	Farina
Egg	1	Soft cooked egg
Bread	1 slice	Enriched white toast
Fat	2 teaspoons	Butter or margarine
Milk	½ cup	Whole milk
Beverage	1 cup	Coffee
Sugar	1 tablespoon	Sugar
LUNCH		
Meat or substitute	3 oz.	Ground chicken
Potato or substitute	1 small	Baked potato (no skin)
Vegetable	½ cup	Pureed asparagus
Fruit	½ cup	Canned cherries
Bread	1	Soft roll
Fat	2 teaspoons	Butter or margarine
Milk	1 cup	Whole milk
Beverage	1 cup	Tea
Sugar	2 teaspoons	Sugar
DINNER		
Soup	½ cup	Cream of mushroom
Meat or substitute	3 oz.	Ground beef
Potato or substitute	1	Mashed potato
Vegetable	½ cup	Pureed or diced carrots
Dessert	1 slice	Vanilla ice cream
Bread	1 slice	Light rye bread
Fat	2 teaspoons	Butter or margarine
Milk	½ cup	Whole milk
Beverage	1 cup	Coffee
Sugar	2 teaspoons	Sugar
8 P.M.		
Fruit	½ cup	Applesauce

Foods usually avoided are: tough, fibrous meat; whole sliced meat or poultry; whole frankfurters; shrimp or lobster; scallops; all cheese except ricotta, cream cheese and cottage cheese; fried eggs; coarse bread or rolls with seeds; hard rolls; raisins; nuts; raw vegetables; spices the patient finds irritating; raw fruits the patient cannot tolerate.

of developing anemia because of radiation's effect on his bone marrow. In the patient receiving radiation to the pelvic area, where there is a large amount of bone, the risk is greater. That is another reason you should encourage patients like Mrs. F. to eat and take a diet supplement. Radiation to the marrow causes cessation of mitosis, with repopulation taking place in 10 to 14 days. High local doses, however, may produce severe marrow injury so that repopulation never occurs. Always pay close attention to each radiation patient's blood count. We did blood counts on Mrs. F. three times a week and recorded them, so the therapist knew her status at all times.

The skin is vulnerable

During treatment, Mrs. F. developed an acute skin reaction in her umbilical and vulval areas. This is an expected complication which ceases after treatment. The effects of therapy on the skin are perhaps the first complication you'll observe with a radiation patient. These effects are characterized by a radiodermatitis or a radioepithelitis, due to loss of epidermal or epithelial layers, and they occur between 3 to 6 weeks after the start of treatment. The patient may notice a drying of the skin with some scaling, a "dry" reaction, which is what Mrs. F. developed.

As therapy proceeds, some patients experience a "wet" reaction. This is characterized by a weeping of the skin usually because the upper layers have been shed. An inappropriate term for this reaction is a "radiation burn"; it is *not* a burn and you should not treat it as such.

In our hospital a patient with a wet reaction is usually given a rest from therapy and the following course of treatment is started. First, the physician may recommend the application of an antibiotic lotion or a steroid cream and exposure of the site to air. Then, the patient is taught to wash the area at least twice a day, usually by just letting warm water run over it, patting it dry, and applying the prescribed cream. Be sure to follow your own hospital's protocol for skin reactions. (Some hospitals believe that keeping the skin as dry as possible is the best treatment for both dry and wet reactions. They instruct patients not to bathe the treatment site and not to use any creams, lotions, or powders. When a wet reaction occurs, they discontinue therapy and simply prescribe a light coating of A & D Ointment to soothe and help in healing.)

In Mrs. F.'s case, we gave the following instructions: Wash (not scrub) the two affected areas with a mild soap and pat them dry; take Sitz baths at least three times a day in salt water (1 tablespoon salt to 1 quart water); avoid exposing the skin to direct sunlight since it cannot heal itself as well as it could before treatment and could get badly sunburned and infected; don't use heating or electric pads or hot-water bags for the same reason; don't use perfumes, powders or ointments containing alcohol, which might dry out the skin. Instead, apply baby oil three times a day as necessary. (After treatment was completed, she would again be permitted to bathe and powder as she pleased.)

Tissue tolerance

The more rapidly cells divide, the more sensitive to radiation they are. Below you'll find cells listed according to their radiosensitivity, lymphocytes being the most radiosensitive.

1. Lymphocytes
2. Erythroblasts
3. Myeloblasts
4. Epithelial cells
   a. Basal cells of the testes
   b. Basal cells of the intestinal crypts
   c. Basal cells of the ovaries
   d. Basal cells of the skin
   e. Basal cells of the secretory glands
   f. Alveolar cells of the lungs and bile ducts
5. Endothelial cells
6. Connective tissue cells
7. Tubular cells of the kidneys
8. Bone cells
9. Nerve cells
10. Brain cells
11. Muscle cells

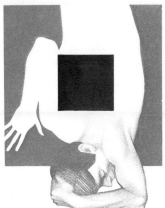

We told her to continue the Sitz baths and start irrigation with a saline solution to her umbilicus during the 1-week rest period. When treatment resumed, the therapist ordered a vulval block applied to prevent further breakdown. Mrs. F. completed treatment after 8 weeks and returned to the follow-up clinic 1 month later with no complaints.

Radiation and other cancers

Radiation may cause other side effects, depending on the area of the body treated. Take the case of Mr. D., a 26-year-old man with diagnosed Stage IIA nodular sclerosing Hodgkin's disease. Mr. D. was post-staging laparotomy with the disease found only above the diaphragm. He was scheduled for external radiation to an extended mantle port for a total of 4000 rads tumor dose.

Some of the preventive measures for Mr. D. were the same as those taken with Mrs. F., since anorexia, nausea, and vomiting might also be expected (see Chapter 16). He did, in fact, develop nausea, which was controlled with prochlorperazine (Compazine), the drug of choice in our department (given either orally or by suppository).

But radiation to the chest can cause different complications, namely significant changes to the lungs and heart. The heart is only affected if the whole heart is included in the treatment area. When that happens, the patient may develop myocarditis or pericarditis, usually 6 months to 1 year after treatment. Suspect myocarditis when you see these symptoms in a patient: precordial pain, tachycardia, weakness, and fever. When a patient develops pericarditis, he displays these signs: shortness of breath on exertion, swelling of the abdomen (with little or no swelling of the feet), fatigue, and cough. Both of these conditions, if they occur, are usually treated by surgical intervention through a pericardial window.

Radiation to the pulmonary system can cause pneumonitis. The tissue tolerance of the lungs is about 2500 rads and if exceeded, the incidence of pneumonitis is increased, but only if more than 25 percent of the pulmonary volume is affected. A patient receiving large doses to large areas of the lung, such as a patient with bronchogenic cancer, is most susceptible.

In caring for a patient getting radiation to the pulmonary system, you should be alert for signs of pneumonitis — a persistent, hacking cough, fever, dyspnea, and weakness.

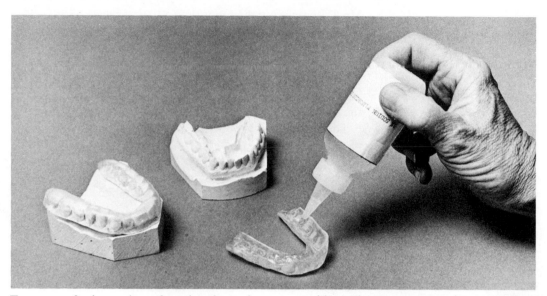

Treatment for it consists of putting the patient on steroids, and rest from therapy. Late effects are fibrosis of the treated lung area, which will be visible on the patient's chest X-rays for the rest of his life.

Mr. D.'s port didn't include large areas of the lungs but did include almost the entire heart. We told him about the possibility of developing either myocarditis or pericarditis. As it turned out, he developed neither.

A problem with teeth

Since Mr. D.'s port extended up to the base of his brain, we sent him to the dentist for preventive care, as we do with all extended-mantle patients. These patients may develop problems because they receive about 4000 rad irradiation to the lower jaw; however, the problems are less severe than those having head and neck irradiation.

Badly decayed teeth should be pulled, and the remaining teeth watched carefully. Irradiation to the salivary glands reduces gland activity, with a resulting decrease in the amount of saliva produced and a reduction of the normal pH. The resulting thick, scanty mucus is less effective in helping to prevent cavities. Why? Because food isn't well diluted, acids aren't well buffered and diluted, and food particles around the teeth aren't washed away as effectively. Advise patients like

The whole tooth
To protect a patient's teeth from the harmful effects of radiation, the dentist forms fluoride carriers from a mold of the patient's teeth. When filled with a 1% sodium fluoride dental gel and fitted in the patient's mouth, these carriers protect all the tooth surfaces.

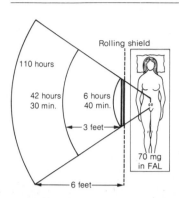

An inside job
In addition to external radiation from machines, patients can receive radiotherapy through topical or internal applications. Radioactive materials can be applied directly to the skin, for example, or implanted in the form of needles, seeds, wires, or catheters directly into the tumor. Implants with a long half-life may be removed after achieving their desired effect, but those with a short half-life may remain in place permanently.

When working around patients with radiation implants, you should give routine care. But keep your exposure to the radiation to a minimum. The figure above shows safe time and distances if you're protected by a lead shield. If you don't have the protection of a shield, though, you should spend considerably less time near the patient. If he has only a 15 mg Ra Eq (radium equivalent) implant, for instance, you can safely spend 3 hours and 10 minutes at the bedside or up to 51 hours 6 feet away. If he has a powerful 90 mg Ra Eq implant, though, you should spend less than ½ hour at the bedside or less than 8½ hours 6 feet away.

Mr. D. to rinse out their mouth 5 to 10 times daily with a salt or peroxide solution.

Radiation decay occurs 1 to 3 years after treatment and can result in crown amputation. Infected teeth usually lead to bone necrosis because the metabolism is affected by the damage to blood vessels feeding the jaw. Thus, you must also reinforce the principles of continued good oral hygiene in these patients.

The dental regime for Mr. D. included prophylactic cleaning of all tooth surfaces and gingival crevices. He was also fitted with fluoride carriers to surround the tooth surfaces, and used a topical fluoride for 5 minutes a day after brushing. No complications developed following this regime.

Hair and spine
Mr. D. lost some hair on his face and the back of his head. This was attributed to change in the rapidly developing epithelial cells around growing hair. The more rapidly the hair grows, the more sensitive the hair follicle. In order of decreasing sensitivity are scalp, male beard, eyebrows, axilla, pubis, and body hair. The hair may grow again, but never at its former rate or density. Mr. D. also developed a wet reaction in his axilla, which was treated with rest from radiotherapy.

Included also within the extended mantle port was Mr. D.'s cervical spine. Spinal-cord tolerance is about 4000 rads. If this is exceeded, two types of injury may result: first, an early, transient myelopathy characterized by paresthesia; second, a later, irreversible injury terminating in paresis or paralysis.

The onset of these complications usually is heralded by the patient complaining of a sensation resembling an electric shock running down his back and over his extremities. This is Lhermitte's sign and can appear several months after treatment. To prevent any such damage, a 50-percent block was placed on Mr. D.'s cervical spine. He completed treatment and is now being followed in hematology-oncology clinic with no evidence of late complications.

The precautions taken with Mr. D. point up the fact that reactions to radiation therapy occur *only* in the areas treated. But if chemotherapy is given in conjunction with radiation therapy, reactions may occur sooner and be more severe. If you are caring for a patient on combined therapy, you should be aware of how the two modalities interact and whether one enhances the other.

5

Chemotherapy: A systemic approach

BY NANCY BURNS, RN, MS

THESE DAYS YOUR CHANCES of caring for a cancer patient receiving chemotherapy are far greater than they were even 2 or 3 years ago. As chemotherapy prolongs life for more patients, even cures patients, more doctors use this treatment. And as more doctors use it, more nurses are called upon to care for the patients.

But, of course, how well a patient does on chemotherapy depends in part on how well you understand this treatment. For instance, you have to know the difference between expected side effects and dangerous toxicities. You have to know the difference between emotional reactions to having cancer and the effects of the drugs themselves. And you have to know what drug protocol and doses a patient should get. With that understanding, you can help the patient cope with the uncomfortable effects of chemotherapy — and maintain his hope in its beneficial effects.

Destroying the doublings
Ideally, the goal of chemotherapy is to cure the patient of his cancer, and to do this, every cancer cell in his body must be destroyed. Accomplishing this goal is a very complex process.

You'll find a good description of how cancer cells multiply in Chapter 2 of this book. The purpose of chemotherapy is to interfere with these cell doublings and, optimally, to destroy all cancer cells. A given dose of an antineoplastic agent always destroys a constant fraction of cells, not a fixed number. This is because only a given percent of cancer cells are dividing when the drug is given. (Most antineoplastic agents can damage cells only during the process of dividing.)

To effectively eradicate a malignant tumor, you must administer either very large doses of antineoplastic agents or start treatment when the number of cells is small enough to allow tumor destruction at reasonably tolerated doses. Until recently, chemotherapy was given only as a last resort — after surgery and radiotherapy had failed. This meant that it wasn't administered to the patient until large numbers of cancer cells already inhabited his body, thereby decreasing the possibility of effective treatment and requiring larger drug doses that produced more severe side effects.

Unfortunately some physicians still don't offer cancer patients the alternative of beginning chemotherapy early. But in progressive cancer treatment centers, chemotherapy is used as adjuvant therapy with surgery or radiotherapy early in the course of the disease.

Which drug, when, and how much?

Choosing the right drug for a cancer patient poses a real challenge to the attending physician, because he must consider so many factors in his decision. For example, what type of cancer does the patient have? An antineoplastic's effectiveness can vary from one cancer to another. Sometimes, the best way to kill certain cancer cells with antineoplastic drugs is to combine several of them, each one chosen to attack a different phase of cell production. When a physician combines drugs, he hopes for synergism, a combined effect greater than the sum of their individual effects.

In some types of cancer, such as acute leukemia, some antineoplastics do well in inducing a remission, but they can't maintain it. So when a patient goes into remission, his doctor may switch to other antineoplastic agents that can't induce a remission, but can maintain it. That's why drugs are often used sequentially to treat a particular type of cancer.

A tumor's location greatly influences the selection of an

TABLE 1. NEOPLASTIC DISEASES THAT RESPOND TO CHEMOTHERAPY

TYPE OF CANCER	USEFUL DRUGS	RESULTS
Prolonged survival or cure		
Gestational trophoblastic tumors	Methotrexate, Dactinomycin, Vinblastine, cis-Platinum	70% cured
Burkitt's tumor	Cyclophosphamide	50% cured
Testicular tumors (seminoma)	Cyclophosphamide with radiotherapy	90-95% respond, 50-60% cured
Wilms' tumor	Dactinomycin with surgery and radiotherapy, Vincristine	30-40% cured (advanced stage) 80-90% cured (early stage)
Neuroblastoma	Cyclophosphamide, Adriamycin, Procarbazine, Vincristine with surgery and/or with radiotherapy	Over 50% respond (advanced stage) Up to 80% long term survival depending on stage
Acute lymphoblastic leukemia	Daunorubicin*, Prednisone*, Vincristine*, 6-Mercaptopurine*, Methotrexate*, BCNU*, L-asparaginase	90% remission; 70% survive beyond 5 years
Hodgkin's disease Stage IIB, IIIB & IV	HN2*, Vincristine*, Prednisone*, Procarbazine*, Bleomycin, Adriamycin, DTIC, Vinblastine	70% respond, 40% survive beyond 5 years
Palliation and prolongation of life		
Prostate carcinoma	estrogens, castration	70% respond with some prolongation of life
Breast carcinoma	androgens, estrogens, alkylating agent*, 5-Fluorouracil*, Vincristine*, Prednisone*, Methotrexate*, Adriamycin, Nafoxidine, Tamoxifen	60-80% respond with probable prolongation of life
Chronic lymphocytic leukemia and Lymphosarcoma	Prednisone, alkylating agents	50% respond with probable prolongation of life
Acute myeloblastic leukemia	Ara-C, Thioguanine, Prednisone, Daunorubicin	65% remission with prolongation of life
Soft tissue and Osteogenic sarcoma	Adriamycin, Methotrexate-CF	20% respond
Palliation with uncertain prolongation of life		
Chronic granulocytic leukemia	alkylating agents, 6-Mercaptopurine, Hydroxyurea	90% respond with good control during most of course
Multiple myeloma	alkylating agents, Prednisone, BCNU, Vincristine	60% respond
Ovary	alkylating agents, cis-Platinum	30-40% respond
Endometrium	progestins	25% respond
Uncertain palliation		
Lung	alkylating agents	30-40% respond briefly
Head and neck	alkylating agents, Methotrexate, Bleomycin, cis-Platinum	20-30% respond briefly
Large bowel	5-Fluorouracil, Ara-C, Mitomycin C, MeCCNU	30-50% respond
Stomach	5-Fluorouracil, Ara-C, Mitomycin C	30% respond
Pancreas and liver	5-Fluorouracil	less than 10% respond
Cervix	alkylating agents, Bleomycin	20% respond
Melanoma	alkylating agents, Vinblastine, DTIC, MeCCNU	20% respond

*May be used in combination.

Adapted from Irwin H. Krakoff, MD, and the American Cancer Society

antineoplastic agent, since drug distribution to the tumor area will determine the antineoplastic's effectiveness. Tumors in bone or in the brain pose particular problems; drug perfusion to bone is poor, and the blood-brain barrier frequently prevents drug entry to the brain.

Other drugs may also interfere with an antineoplastic's effectiveness by competing for protein binding sites (thus altering the anticipated blood level of the cancer drug and increasing the risk of side effects). Some doctors feel that antinauseants, for example, may reduce the effectiveness of an antineoplastic through drug interaction.

What factors does a physician consider when he decides dosage and timing in a chemotherapeutic drug? Well, first he considers the margin between a therapeutic dose and a toxic dose. This is very narrow in antineoplastics. So the attending physician always calculates doses with great accuracy, basing them on body surface area and kilograms of body weight. Standard doses for individual drugs, of course, may be altered in combination therapy.

Second, he considers the time that must lapse between doses to allow recovery of normal cells. He must calculate this time lapse carefully, since the tumor cells begin to regrow during it. And if the normal cells recover slowly, the tumor may regrow to pretreatment levels or greater, eventually killing the patient.

Third, the doctor has to consider the side effects of each drug and when they're most likely to occur. The most common side effect is damage to rapidly growing normal cells, including cells in the bone marrow, hair follicles, and the mucous lining of the GI tract. Of these, the most serious is damage to cells in the bone marrow, which can depress white cells, platelets, and red cells.

The time of the most severe depression is called the nadir. But the nadir for platelets may occur at a different time than the nadir for white cells. That's why multiple drug therapy can be so complex; the doctor has to choose drugs with different side effects or side effects that occur at different times.

If your patient is on multiple drug therapy, as most patients on chemotherapy are, you should keep a flow chart of laboratory data so you can pinpoint the nadir for each blood component and how long it takes the patient to recover from bone marrow depression. This will help you anticipate possible complications, such as infection and bleeding, so you can treat them early.

Finally, since most antineoplastics are metabolized in the liver and excreted by the kidneys, he must consider the patient's liver and kidney function.

Once the doctor settles on the right drug therapy for a patient, monitoring its effects — and even administering the therapy — may rest in your hands.

Along the baseline

As you can imagine, antineoplastic drugs are stressors. And, a patient's tolerance to stressors depends on his physiologic status. So, before administering antineoplastic agents, you should make a careful nursing assessment to establish a baseline against which to measure your patient's progress.

You should assess:

• *Nutritional status*. Check his weight, muscle tone, and skin turgor.

• *Skin condition*. Examine carefully for skin lesions, incisions, or wounds; remember that antineoplastics interfere with cell growth necessary to wound healing. Also check for infections, which could increase metabolic activity and decrease the patient's tolerance for chemotherapy.

• *Oral condition*. Check for oral irritation, bleeding gums, ill-fitting dentures, or poor oral hygiene. Disseminated cancer frequently results in anorexia and rapid weight loss, which cause changes in oral mucosa, such as decreased salivation and poorly functioning oral mucosa.

• *Degree of mobility*. Evaluate how much activity he can participate in before he becomes fatigued. Does he show an increase in respiration or other indications of hypoxia with exertion?

• *Psychological status*. Familiarizing yourself with your patient's personality, his emotional state, and his relationships with family members will help you evaluate any psychological changes. Various emotional reactions, such as fear, depression, and denial may result from the patient's attempts to cope with his disease. But to deal effectively with emotional reactions, you must be able to distinguish them from the psychological changes produced by the chemotherapy itself. One of our patients, for instance, became quite euphoric after beginning therapy with prednisone. We might have called in a

Common protocols

OAP *(Regulated according to the degree of bone marrow depression)*
Vincristine (Oncovin): 1.4 mg/m² I.V. push on day 1
Cytarabine (Ara-C): 200 mg/m² per day for 5 days as continuous I.V. infusion
Prednisone: 100 mg total dose daily (25 mg q.i.d.) for 5 days

POMP *(Regulated according to the degree of bone marrow depression)*
6-Mercaptopurine (Purinethol): 500 mg/m² per day for 5 days
Vincristine (Oncovin): 1.4 mg/m² I.V. push on days 1 and 7
Methotrexate: 7.5 mg/m² I.V. daily for 5 days
Prednisone: 100 mg per day (25 mg q.i.d.) for 5 days

COMFU-P *(repeated monthly)*
Cyclophosphamide (Cytoxan): 120 mg/m² I.V. per day for 5 days
Vincristine (Oncovin): 0.625 mg/m² I.V. push on days 1 and 5
Methotrexate: 4 mg/m² I.V. per day for 5 days
Fluorouracil (5-FU): 180 mg/m² I.V. per day for 5 days
Prednisone: 40 mg/m² per day in divided doses for 5 days

CODFU *(repeated monthly)*
Cyclophosphamide (Cytoxan): 120 mg/m² I.V. per day for 5 days
Vincristine (Oncovin): 0.625 mg/m² I.V. push on days 1 and 5
Dactinomycin (Actinomycin D): 0.25 mg I.V. per day for 5 days
Fluorouracil (5-FU): 180 mg/m² I.V. per day for 5 days

psychiatric consultant if we hadn't known that euphoria is a common side effect of prednisone. Methotrexate, on the other hand, can cause malaise, and vincristine sulfate (Oncovin) can trigger depression, a state so common in cancer patients it's difficult to recognize as drug-related.

Since laboratory tests (blood counts, bone marrow aspirations, and so on) and X-rays can paint a picture of a patient's progress, record the results and know what they mean in relation to the patient and his treatment. Also record the patient's drug protocol on his flow sheet. Protocols are drugs commonly given together on a set schedule. The day of the first dose is called Day One. Each day after that is numbered in sequence with the nadir for each drug expected to occur near a specifically numbered day. When a drug regimen is repeated, it again starts on Day One.

A double-check pays

Naturally you know to check the drug label to make sure it's what the doctor ordered; you'd do that with any medication. But with antineoplastic drugs, you'd be wise to double-check, since several drugs — for example, 5FC and 5FU; BCNU and CCNU — have very similar names. Check the physician's order sheet, not just a medication card — and be sure to check the dose too. Fatal mistakes can occur.

If the drug is to be administered intravenously, also be sure to check the method of administration. Some are given I.V. push; some are mixed with a specific amount of solution; some are administered only into an already established free-flowing I.V. infusion; and some are administered by I.V. drip at a specified rate.

Monitor I.V. infusion carefully, since too rapid an infusion may cause severe toxic effects. Some drugs, particularly mechlorethamine hydrochloride and doxorubicin hydrochloride, cause severe local tissue damage if extravasation occurs. If you see signs of extravasation, notify the physician immediately so he can lessen local tissue damage. If the I.V. infiltrates and you have to restart it, do so quickly to avoid lowering the blood level of the drug.

If vomiting occurs after oral administration, notify the physician. Why? Not only because it can be a sign of toxicity with some drugs, but also because the patient will be losing all or part of his drug dose. The physician will have to alter the chemotherapy to account for it. For the same reason, you should notify the physician if the patient misses a dose for some reason or if his dose is delayed.

The good, the bad, and the ugly

Perhaps more than any other person, you're in a good position to keep track of the chemotherapy's effects — good or bad.

X-rays, of course, will show exact changes in tumor size. But sometimes you can actually see that the tumor has gotten smaller. And even if you can't see changes in the tumor itself, you can look for signs of progress: better appetite, weight gain, greater mobility, higher tolerance for exercise, and improved breathing.

At the same time that chemotherapy is working, though, it most likely will cause uncomfortable side effects. Because it is rapidly breaking down cancer cells, which then enter the circulatory system and exit via the kidneys, it may affect the patient's kidney function. Watch out for an elevated BUN. Be sure to keep accurate intake-output records, too. Remember that hyperuricemia, coupled with decreased food intake, can sap a patient's energy. To speed excretion of uric acid and decrease the hazard of crystal and urate stone formation, increase the patient's fluid intake.

Occasionally the doctor will order allopurinol (Zyloprim) to lower uric acid levels. If he orders it for a patient on mercaptopurine (Purinethol), be sure the mercaptopurine dosage is reduced to ⅓ or ¼ the usual dose. Allopurinol blocks the enzyme responsible for detoxifying mercaptopurine, so it can cause toxic blood levels of mercaptopurine if the mercaptopurine is given in the usual dose.

Nausea, vomiting, and anorexia occur frequently during chemotherapy. They are serious problems, not only because they are very frustrating to the patient but also because they affect his tolerance to food at a time when he needs nutrients to maintain cellular function. Severe vomiting may cause fluid and electrolyte imbalances. Loss of hydrogen and chloride may result in hypochloremic alkalosis.

By providing small, nutritious snacks and planning meal schedules to meet his best tolerance times, you can help him. If possible, arrange his main meal for early morning, or give him small servings of food throughout the day. You may have difficulty arranging such special treatment with the dietary department, but your patient will appreciate your efforts and

Common protocols

MOPP *(repeated every 28 days)*
Mechlorethamine (nitrogen mustard): 6 mg/m² I.V. push on days 1 and 8
Vincristine (Oncovin): 1.4 mg/m² I.V. push on days 1 and 8
Procarbazine (Matulane): 100 mg/m² per day P.O. for 10 days
Prednisone: 40 mg/m² per day P.O. for 10 days

COP *(repeated every 15 days)*
Cyclophosphamide (Cytoxan): 800 mg/m² I.V. push on day 1
Vincristine (Oncovin): 1.4 mg/m² on day 1
Prednisone: 100 mg total daily dose (25 mg q.i.d.) for five days

MAC *(repeated every 21 days)*
Methotrexate: 4 mg/m² I.V. per day for 5 days
Dactinomycin (Actinomycin D): 0.5 mg I.V. per day for 5 days
Cyclophosphamide (Cytoxan): 120 mg/m² I.V. per day for 5 days

COAP *(Regulated according to the degree of bone marrow depression)*
Cyclophosphamide (Cytoxan): 100 mg/m² per day I.V. for 5 days
Vincristine (Oncovin): 1.4 mg/m² as I.V. push on day 1
Cytarabine (Ara-C): 100 mg/m² per day for 5 days as continuous I.V. infusion
Prednisone: 100 mg total daily dose (25 mg q.i.d.) for 5 days

CANCER CHEMOTHERAPEUTIC AGENTS

AGENTS	ROUTE	USUAL ADULT DOSE	ASSOCIATED SIDE EFFECTS
Alkylating Agents			
Mechlorethamine HCl (HN2, Mustargen)	I.V.	0.4 mg/kg single or divided doses	Moderate to severe depression of peripheral blood cell count and bone marrow. Leukopenia, thrombo-cytopenia, bleeding. Toxicity often delayed 2-3 weeks after last dose. Alopecia and hemorrhagic cystitis occur occasionally with cyclophosphamide, N&V Myelosuppression and renal toxicity may occur with lomustine.
Chlorambucil (Leukeran)	Oral	0.1-0.2 mg/kg/day 6-12 mg/day	
Melphalan (Alkeran)	Oral	0.1 mg/kg/day x 7 2.4 mg/day maintenance	
Triethylenethiophosphoramide (TSPA, Thiotepa)	Intratumor / I.V.	45-60 mg initially repeated weekly depending on blood count / ½ local dose at 1-4 week intervals	
Busulfan (Myleran)	Oral	2-6 mg/day	
Cyclophosphamide (Cytoxan)	Oral / I.V.	1-5 mg/kg/day / 10-15 mg/kg every 7-10 days	
Lomustine (CCNU)	Oral	100-300 mg/day	
Pipobroman (Vercyte)	Oral	1.5-2.5 mg/kg/day	
Uracil Mustard* (Uracil Mustard)	Oral	0.5 mg/kg/day	
Antimetabolites			
Methotrexate (Methotrexate)	Oral / I.V. / I.M.	2.5-5.0 mg/day / 25-50 mg 1-2x weekly / 15-30 mg/day for 5 days	Oral and GI tract ulcerations, bone marrow depression with leukopenia, thrombocytopenia, and bleeding. With large doses or overdoses, Leucovorin (C.F. rescue) for neutralization of toxic effects is necessary
6-Mercaptopurine (6-MP, Purinethol)	Oral	2.5 mg/kg/day	Bone marrow depression with excessive doses
6-Thioguanine (6-TG, Thioguanine, Lanvis)	Oral	2.0-3.0 mg/kg/day	
5-Fluorouracil (5-FU, Fluorouracil, Efudex)	I.V.	12 mg/kg/day x 3 Smaller dose, 1-2 x weekly for maintenance	Stomatitis, nausea, GI injury, bone marrow depression
Floxuridine (FUDR)*		0.1-0.6 mg/kg/day	Bone marrow depression, megaloblastosis, leukopenia, thrombocytopenia, N&V
Cytarabine (Ara-C, Cytosar)	I.V.	1.0-3.0 mg/kg/day x 10-20 days	
Antibiotics			
Doxorubicin HCl (Adriamycin)	I.V.	50-75 mg/m² in single or divided doses every 3 weeks	Stomatitis, N&V, alopecia, bone marrow depression. Cardiac toxicity at cumulative doses over 500 mg/m²
Bleomycin (Blenoxane)	I.V., I.M. S.C.	0.25 units/kg/day x 5-7 Maintenance 1.0-2.0 mg/day	Mucous membrane ulcerations, alopecia, possible pulmonary fibrosis
Mithramycin (Mithracin)	I.V.	25 micrograms/kg every other day x 3-4	Bone marrow depression particularly thrombocytopenia, bleeding, hypocalcemia, hepatic toxicity at large doses, N&V

CANCER CHEMOTHERAPEUTIC AGENTS

AGENTS	ROUTE	USUAL ADULT DOSE	ASSOCIATED SIDE EFFECTS
Mitomycin C (Mutamycin)	I.V.	20 mg/m² I.V. once or 2 mg/m²/day for 10 days	Bone marrow depression, N&V
Dactinomycin (Actinomycin D, Cosmegen)	I.V.	0.5 mg/day for 5 days	Soft tissue necrosis with extravasation, various anemias, N&V
Steroid Compounds			
Polyestradiol phosphate (Estradurin)	I.M.	40 mg I.M. every 2-4 weeks	Fluid retention, N&V, feminization and gynecomastia in men, masculinization in women, weight gain, acne, uterine bleeding, increased libido
Diethylstibestrol diphosphate (Stiphostrol, Stibilium)	I.V. Oral	0.5-1 gm in 300 ml PSS 150-600 mg/day	
Medroxyprogesterone acetate (Depo-Provera)	I.M.	400-1000 mg per week	
Megestrol acetate (Megace)	Oral	160-320 mg/day for 2 months	
Testolactone (Teslac)	Oral I.M.	1 gm/day 100 mg 3 times/week	
Calusterone (Methosarb)	Oral	150-300 mg/day	
Dromostanolone propionate (Drolban)	I.M.	100 mg 3 times/week	
Prednisone	Oral	15-100 mg/day	Fluid retention, GI bleeding psychiatric changes, diabetes osteoporosis
Miscellaneous Drugs			
L-Asparaginase (Elspar, Kidrolase)	I.V.	200-1000 IU/kg 3-7x weekly for 28 days	Anorexia, N&V, weight loss. Somnolence, lethargy, confusion. Hypoproteinemia (including albumin and fibrinogen.) Hypolipidemia and/or hyperlipidemia, abnormal liver function tests, fatty liver. Azotemia. Granulocytopenia, lymphopenia, thrombocytopenia (usually mild and transient), and anaphalaxis.
Procarbazine HCl (Matulane, MIH, Natulan)	Oral	50-300 mg/day	Bone marrow depression with leukopenia and thrombocytopenia, mental depression, N&V
Vinblastine sulfate (Velban, V.L.B., Velbe)	I.V.	0.1-0.2 mg/kg weekly	Alopecia, areflexia, bone marrow depression, N&V
Vincristine sulfate (Oncovin, VCR)	I.V.	0.015-0.05 mg/kg weekly	Areflexia, muscular weakness, peripheral neuritis, paralytic ileus, mild bone marrow depression
cis-Platinum*	I.V.	1-3 mg/kg/week	Deafness, renal tubular damage, intractable N&V
Dacarbazine DTIC (DTIC)	I.V.	2-4.5 mg/kg/day for 10 days	Depression, N&V
Mitotane (Lysodren)	Oral	9-10 gm/day	
Quinacrine HCl (Atabrine)	Intrapleural Intraperitoneal	200-1000 mg per infusion	Paralytic ileus, peritoneal or pleural pain
Hydroxyrea* (Hydrea)	Oral	20-30 mg/kg/day	Bone marrow depression
Nitrosourea (BCNU, Carmustine)	I.V.	100-400 mg/day	Myelosuppression, renal toxicity, N&V

*Not available in Canada

Adapted from Irwin H. Krakoff, MD, and the American Cancer Society

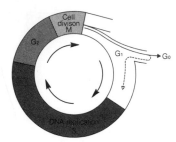

How antineoplastic agents work
Antineoplastic drugs stop cancer cell production by interrupting protein synthesis, thereby preventing such cells from reproducing and surviving.

Each of the many cell proteins is manufactured at a specific point within the cell cycle, which is divided into several stages: Phase G_1 is the period before DNA synthesis (at which time the cell may also become dormant, a state designated G_0); Phase S represents DNA synthesis; Phase G_2 includes RNA synthesis; and Phase M represents mitosis, including prophase, metaphase, anaphase, and telophase. The duration of any cell's life cycle differs according to the tissue of origin, but the average length of the process, excluding mitosis, is 10 hours.

Antineoplastic agents may be either cell cycle specific or nonspecific. Cell cycle specific antineoplastics are the antimetabolites, which act at Phase S, and the plant alkaloids, which attack at Phase M. The alkylating agents are all cell cycle nonspecific and can act at all phases of the cell cycle.

Repeated administration of one antineoplastic agent tends to develop resistant cancer cells so that alternate drugs must be substituted. In fact, the success of any chemotherapeutic program depends on the extent to which drugs may be combined in therapy.

any concessions you gain. One of our patients, who was anorexic during the day, was always hungry around midnight, so at that time we fed him meals his family provided.

If a patient develops a dietary deficiency from chemotherapy, get him some dietary supplements and ask the dietitian to add more calories to his menu. Freezing the supplements and serving them like ice cream in sundaes and shakes makes them more palatable.

Stomatitis, an early sign of toxicity, may be a severe problem. But if you give your patient proper mouth care before stomatitis develops, you may prevent it or decrease its severity. Apply hydrogen peroxide and water directly to his oral mucosa, or use it as a mouth rinse followed by a coating of substrate of milk of magnesia. Try one or both of these every 4 hours around the clock. When more than 6 hours pass without mouth care, mucosal deterioration begins. (To make substrate of milk of magnesia, discard the clear liquid at the top of the bottle and use the thick, white material that remains.) Never use lemon juice and glycerine, since these substances decrease saliva, change the mouth's pH, and dry the oral mucosa. Teach and encourage your patient to care for his own mouth, so he will be more independent when he leaves the hospital.

Is he uncomfortable eating? Before meals, give him a mouth swish of lidocaine hydrochloride (Xylocaine Viscous) to anesthetize his oral mucosa. Always examine his mouth daily for early signs of stomatitis. Tell him to report bleeding gums or a burning sensation when he drinks acid liquids. Also order a bland diet for him.

Diarrhea or abdominal cramps often indicate hypermotility of the intestinal tract due to cellular damage. Report them to the physician promptly, remembering that the frequency of the episodes indicates the extent of tissue destruction. Diarrhea sometimes leads to electrolyte imbalance and dehydration and eventual acidosis. To prevent this, the physician may order a bland or low-residue diet, high in constipating foods. If the patient has anal tenderness, you should apply A & D ointment.

Drug therapy also can damage blood forming organs, decreasing red cells, white cells, and platelets. Your patient may get tired easily, develop infections, and bleed abnormally.

Suppression of white cells decreases a patient's defense

against infection, so be careful to wash your hands when caring for him. Daily blood studies and bone marrow aspirations provide an accurate patient profile. If your patient develops a fever, report it immediately and search for its cause. Leukopenia or massive systemic infections of *Candida* and *Pseudomonas* occur in many patients and cause death in a few hours, if not treated aggressively.

A decrease in platelets may make a patient bleed abnormally from minor trauma such as needle punctures, shaving cuts, and bruises. Warn him about this when you examine him. Observe his stools, vomitus, and urine for color changes that indicate organ bleeding. And protect him against tissue injury by using soft toothbrushes and padding his bony prominences. If he already has tissue injury, you may have to discontinue I.M. injections and give platelet transfusions.

Patients may have a transfusion reaction or develop hepatitis if transfusions are frequent. Sometimes, though, you can't tell if liver damage is caused by tumor invasion, hepatitis, or a toxic drug reaction. You must know an antineoplastic's side effects, including the rare ones listed in the company's literature. Remember the following:

• Nitrogen mustard or procarbazine can cause convulsions.

• Doxorubicin hydrochloride (Adriamycin) can cause heart damage progressing to congestive heart failure. Carefully monitor the patient receiving Adriamycin for fluid retention and changes in cardiac output, rate, and rhythm.

• Bleomycin can cause changes in respiratory function and even pulmonary fibrosis.

• Vincristine causes neural damage. Neural changes in the patient's lower gastrointestinal tract usually result in severe constipation. Manage constipation carefully with a high-fiber diet, stool softeners, and possibly suppositories to prevent impactions and obstruction. Remember to ask the patient on Vincristine to report tingling, numbness, and tremors in his extremities, since these are early signs of neural drug damage. By the time the patient has trouble heel-walking or getting out of chairs, the damage is severe. The drug is discontinued, though the side effects can remain as long as 2 years.

Of all the side effects of chemotherapy, alopecia can be the most distressing to many patients. Antineoplastics damage hair follicles as much as, if not more than, malignant cells. So a patient may lose some or all of his hair, including scalp hair,

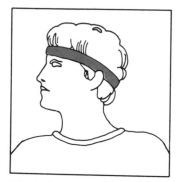

Alleviating alopecia
By cutting off the blood supply to
the hair follicles, scalp
tourniquets protect the patient's
hair from the damaging effects of
chemotherapy. You can use a
wide Penrose drain, or a
pneumatic tourniquet placed as
above. A pneumatic tourniquet is
more convenient because you
can adjust the pressure during a
long I.V. infusion of a drug.

eyebrows, eyelashes, and underarm and pubic hair. Warn
your patient about this possibility. But reassure him that it will
regrow in about 8 weeks after therapy, though possibly in a
different texture and color. You might introduce him to
another chemotherapy patient whose hair has regrown, just to
set his mind at rest. Often, you can minimize scalp hair loss by
applying a scalp tourniquet during I.V. administration. This
protects the hair from high concentrations of the drug. For
best results, keep the tourniquet in place for 10 to 15 minutes.

Knowing when to stop
Every physician must wrestle with the decision of when to
discontinue therapy — because of either destruction of all
cancer cells, drug resistance, or severe drug toxicity.

Since no one can tell for sure when all cancer cells have been
destroyed, the decision to discontinue therapy can be difficult
even when a patient has achieved a prolonged remission. For
example, suppose a patient has been receiving chemotherapy
for two years with no clinical signs of tumor. Can the physician
safely discontinue treatment and assume all the cancer cells
have been destroyed? Or would discontinuing therapy expose
the patient to the risk of a small number of cancer cells regrow-
ing, and eventually killing him? In short, which is more risky:
continued side effects, or discontinuing therapy?

To avoid this dilemma, many chemotherapeutic regimens
are set to last only a specified length of time. No matter what
the patient's condition, though, the end of therapy may be
disconcerting to him; he may worry that his cancer will return
without the intervention of these life-saving drugs. Explain
that the doctor will closely follow his progress, seeing him as
often as once or twice a month at first. If any signs of recurrence appear, he can quickly resume therapy. Even if the
remission holds over several years, the doctor will continue
seeing him biannually or annually.

Caring for a cancer patient on chemotherapy can challenge
your nursing skills. You must be able to establish a data base,
assess the patient...and, above all, give the patient emotional
support. Unfortunately, some nurses still don't see the chal-
lenging aspects of cancer nursing. But with your knowledge,
you may be able to change their feelings.

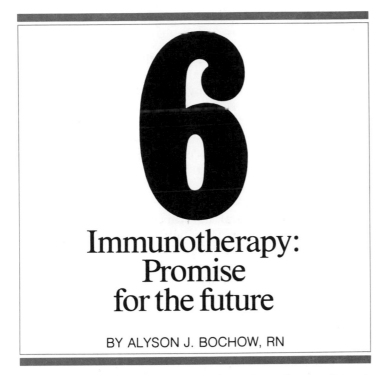

Immunotherapy:
Promise
for the future

BY ALYSON J. BOCHOW, RN

ADMITTEDLY, IMMUNOTHERAPY is an investigational treatment for cancer. Why then should it interest you?

The answer, of course, is that you do care for cancer patients. Many of them find comfort in the hope that cancer research may yet turn up some treatment of value to them. They read about immunotherapy and may want to discuss it with you.

But their questions may not be easy to answer. Many of the significant discoveries of immunology have occurred in the past decade — too recent to have been included in the curriculum when many of you were in school. Even the newer textbooks mention immunotherapy briefly or not at all. So you begin at a disadvantage unless you have kept yourself informed about events at the very forefront of medical research.

Nurses are significantly involved in the clinical research now being pursued so intensively. In most centers they administer immunotherapy. And they are vital contributors to the oncology team, playing an active part in planning and evaluating treatment. In this role, nurses find satisfaction in educating patients and shaping their attitudes toward immunotherapy. Since it is experimental, the patient may feel

Immune, three ways

Immunotherapy divides into three main categories. To answer your patients' questions, you should be familiar with all three:

ACTIVE
Administration of antigen and subsequent development of immunity (antibody) by the host.
Specific
Stimulates immune response to a tumor-associated antigen.
Examples: autologous tumor cells; allogeneic tumor cells; modified tumor cells.
Nonspecific
Stimulates immune response to a wide variety of antigens including tumor-associated antigens.
Examples: BCG (bacillus Calmette-Guerin); C. parvulum (Corynebacterium parvulum); DNCB (2, 4 dinitrochlorobenzene for basal or squamous cell carcinoma); pertussis vaccine; MER (methanol extracted residue of BCG); vaccina; poly Ic; bacterial endotoxins; polynucleotides.
PASSIVE
Direct transfer of transient immunity.
Examples: antisera; lymphocytes; cross-immunization and cross transfusion.
ADOPTIVE
Transfer of immunity (passive) and subsequent development of immunity by host (active).
Examples: Transfer factor; immune RNA.

like the proverbial guinea pig. Even though he may be reluctant to express his anxiety, he intently observes his nurse's attitude, looking to her for confidence. A nurse who is knowledgeable about immunotherapy can alleviate the patient's anxiety. And since most patients are treated as outpatients, they may come in contact with nurses not employed in cancer research. If you should encounter such a patient, you'll want to know at least the rudiments of the exciting developments in this field.

A radical, new theory

In the late 1960s a radical, new cancer theory was proposed. Since then some scientists — but by no means all — have become persuaded of the theory's validity. It states that each of us continually produces cancer cells within our bodies. Why do tumors fail to develop? Because, these scientists say, our immune systems protect us; cancer becomes clinically apparent only when our immune systems cease to function properly. Much of the evidence supporting the theory comes from animal studies, but several clinical observations also support it. Here is a sampling:

• Postoperative patients are commonly found to have cancer cells in circulating blood and operative wound washings — yet many never develop clinically apparent cancer.

• Occasionally a patient will develop rapidly progressing recurrent disease 10 or 20 years after an apparent cure. Some immunological defense system seemingly protected him during the tumor-free interval.

• Patients with congenital or acquired immunologic deficiencies have a much greater incidence of cancer than found in the normal population.

• Renal transplant patients who receive immunosuppressant therapy develop cancer at a rate at least 80 times greater than the general population.

Other experimental evidence not only supports the immune theory but also provides a clinically useful measure of patients' immune capability. With a simple skin test, scientists demonstrated that growing tumors can nonspecifically suppress the immune system. They note that most healthy people can be sensitized to certain chemicals. For instance, over 95% of the normal population will react to 2,4 dinitrochlorobenzene (DNCB). All it takes is 2,000 mcg of the chemical on a small area (20 sq mm) of skin to arouse an immune response. If challenged 14 days later with 100, 50, and 25 mcg of DNCB, a "memory" flare may be produced at the original site — the so-called delayed cutaneous hypersensitivity response.

The DNCB test provides an index of immune function. People with properly functioning immune systems display this secondary response; those with faulty immune systems display no such response and are said to be anergic. When a cancer patient is found to be anergic, experience shows that he usually has a rapidly growing tumor and a poor prognosis. But what would happen if one were able to stimulate the immune system? Would this control the cancer?

Three ways to strengthen immunity

Several different immunotherapeutic modalities are being evaluated currently. They are divided into three general classifications: active, passive, and adoptive immunotherapy.

Active immunotherapy involves injecting an antigen to stimulate the patient's own immune response against cancer, much the same as in vaccination against measles or mumps. The injected substance can be a specific cancer antigen or it can be a nonspecific antigen that produces a general stimulation of the immune system.

Active specific immunotherapy includes vaccination with autologous, allogeneic, or modified tumor vaccine.

The autologous vaccine is produced from the patient's own tumor. Small doses are injected intradermally at various sites in an effort to stimulate the immune mechanism.

The allogeneic vaccine is a mixture of cells of the same type as the patient's. These donor cells may be more immunogenic than the patient's own cells because they introduce antigens new to the patient's immune system — antigens that appear to stimulate the immune system to a greater degree.

The third type of vaccine, modified tumor cells, contains tumor cells treated artificially to increase their antigenicity. One way to do this is to treat tumor cells with neuraminidase, a chemical found to stimulate the immune system. It does so by removing a coating on the tumor cells making them easier to neutralize. The tumor cells are usually first irradiated, a process that stops growth, although live tumor cells have been given in doses too small to allow growth in the recipient.

Tumor cell vaccines are administered in small (approxi-

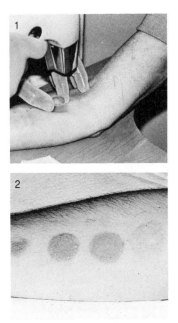

Reading the barometer
In immunotherapy, skin reactions act as a barometer; they can tell you the patient's overall immune capability and how he is reacting to therapy. For instance, after the application of DNCB (Figure 1) skin reactions indicate your patient's immune system. Figure 2 shows a positive response to the DNCB. The patient has developed an immune memory (flare), which you can see in the reaction to the second dose (challenge).

mately 0.1 cc) intradermal injections. You will note that the injection sites become reddened or pruritic and may develop painful ulcerations. Instruct the patient to keep the sites clean. Generally, washing the injection sites twice a day with soap and water is sufficient, but if they should become excoriated, they may be washed with hydrogen peroxide and covered with a dressing. Fever, chills, and general malaise, which may occur after an injection, can usually be controlled with acetaminophen (Tylenol), 2 tablets every 4 to 6 hours as needed.

Nonspecific immunotherapy is used to stimulate the immune system in a different manner. Antigens other than cancer types cause increased antibody and lymphocyte production. Today the most publicized nonspecific agent is BCG. It is the same attenuated bovine *tubercle bacillus* used to immunize patients against tuberculosis.

BCG has proved very effective as local treatment for superficial or subcutaneous metastases of melanoma. In fact, 90% of immunocompetent melanoma patients have complete regressions of their tumor nodules after the nodules were injected with BCG. (Immunocompetency is determined by a positive response to the DNCB skin test described earlier.) In 20% of these patients, even uninjected melanoma nodules regressed, suggesting that BCG produced a systemic reaction as well. However, patients with negative DNCB skin tests responded poorly to the intradermal injections, and no uninjected lesions regressed.

BCG immunotherapy is accomplished by various techniques, including scarification, intradermal injection, and the multiple puncture tine technique. We use the tine technique to administer BCG because it is quicker and causes less discomfort than the alternative, scarification. The tine technique requires a 36-pronged grid square attached to a magnet. First, the BCG is applied to a small area of the skin, and then the tines are pressed through the BCG into the skin. An inflammatory reaction occurs at the injection site after the patient becomes sensitized to BCG and the level of circulating antibodies (both tumor-specific and nonspecific) increases.

When intradermal injection is accomplished by injecting BCG directly into a tumor nodule, the patient may complain of general symptoms — fever, chills, and general malaise — as well as localized abscesses and drainage. By pretreating patients with antihistamines and acetaminophen, these side effects can be decreased. If they persist, isoniazid (INH), 300 mg daily, is effective. These same side effects may also occur after treatment by the tine technique, although they are less severe.

The lymph nodes that drain BCG injection sites sometimes become enlarged and painful, resembling metastases. To differentiate this reactive hyperplasia from metastases may require biopsy. BCG also may cause an elevation in SGOT or alkaline phosphatase levels or the appearance of jaundice — suggesting liver dysfunction. The reaction is usually temporary. In animals excessive doses of BCG have been known to enhance tumor growth. Although this complication is rare in humans, the immune response should be monitored by skin testing to detect any immunosuppressive effects of BCG therapy.

Passive immunotherapy, though still in the early investigational stages, holds promise. It involves the person-to-person transfer of established immunity, either with antibodies or by other immunologically active material or cells. Antitumor antibodies can be transferred from someone who has been cured of his tumor to a patient with a growing cancer. The problem is, other antibodies, in addition to antitumor antibodies, are transferred too, and they may destroy the recipient's normal tissues. To solve this problem, methods for isolating tumor-associated antibodies in sera are currently being developed. Studies have shown that close family members and associates of cancer patients also have high levels of circulating antitumor antibodies; these people too are possible donors of antibody-containing sera (antisera).

Lymphocytes from cured cancer patients could also be used to transfer passive immunity, but the problems are similar. Compatible donors must be found by human leukocyte antigen typing (HLA typing). The donors of the antisera mentioned above could also donate their sensitized lymphocytes. A potentially less risky method would involve using the patient's own lymphocytes. These lymphocytes could be sensitized in the laboratory and reinfused into the patient to increase the lymphocyte-to-tumor cell ratio.

Passive immunotherapy has been accomplished between patients, paired according to blood and tumor type. Tumor from patient A is subcutaneously transplanted to patient B and vice versa; they are cross-immunized. Then blood is removed

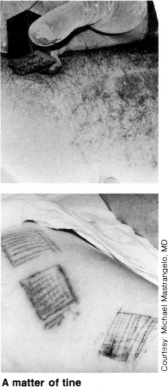

Courtesy: Michael Mastrangelo, MD

A matter of tine
The top picture shows the administration of BCG (bacillus of Calmette and Guerin) by the tine technique. The lower photograph shows the sites of administrations by scarification.

BCG is preserved by freeze-drying and distributed in 1 cc vials, which must be stored in the refrigerator until 1 hour before administration to ensure potency. To prepare the vaccine, dilute the organism with 1 cc of sterile water without preservative. Mix well.

from each patient and separated into red and white cells. The red cells are returned to the donor, while the white cells from patient A, which contain sensitized lymphocytes, are transferred to patient B and vice versa (cross transfusion).

Adoptive immunotherapy involves two steps: The patient first accepts passive immunity and then actively maintains that immunity. For example, the patient's lymphocytes can be stimulated by incubating them with tumor cells, then reinfused into the patient. Adoptive immunotherapy, like passive immunotherapy, transfers immunity directly. Unlike passive immunotherapy (which produces short-lived immunity because lymphocytes are continually made and destroyed), adoptive immunotherapy causes the patient to adopt the immunity as part of his ongoing immunological defense system.

One current form of adoptive immunotherapy involves the transference of informational molecules — for example, extracts of human white cells called transfer factor, or lymphoid extracts from animals called immune RNA, can transfer cellular immunity. Both possess two distinct advantages over passive and adoptive immunotherapy. First, the extract containing instructional molecules carries the immune message, rather than the short-lived lymphocytes. Second, the extract itself is not immunogenic and hence does not contain antigens that might lead to compatibility problems.

The wide variety of treatments currently being investigated provides a challenge for all nurses. We need to understand the rationale for immunotherapy as it applies to cancer if we are to join in implementing its great promise.

SKILLCHECK 1

1. Jerry Cooper is a 16-year-old Hodgkin's disease patient receiving radiation therapy to his chest in an extended mantle port. You have discussed the importance of his diet with Jerry and his mother and warned him to stay out of direct sunlight. Three weeks later, however, you notice that Jerry is losing weight and has developed a skin reaction across his shoulders. Jerry says nothing. His mother, however, complains that he runs around with his friends too much. She says he went to a beach party the previous Sunday and ate pizza. What do you do in this situation?

2. Joseph O'Malley, a retired 68-year-old railroad conductor, has been informed by his physician that he will be discharged from the hospital in two days. He has been a cooperative patient, and his recovery from a mandible resection has been uneventful. Suddenly, Mr. O'Malley becomes very demanding. He is angry if his dinner tray is five minutes late, he calls you to adjust his bed every half hour, and he quarrels with his wife during visiting hours. What can you do?

3. You are prepping the abdomen of Rita Romano, a friendly 32-year-old hotel maid scheduled for a hysterectomy and salpingo-oophorectomy the next morning. She has signed the surgeon's release and understands that he will remove her ovaries. But when you mention menopause to her, she becomes withdrawn. What do you do now?

4. Mary Lou Whitney is a 32-year-old tennis instructor with recurrent malignant melanoma (nodular) on her right thigh. Seven days ago, she was admitted to the hospital for intradermal injections of BCG directly into one of the tumor nodules. This morning, she stops you in the hall outside her room and complains that she has swelling and pain in her right groin. What do you do in this situation?

5. Sara Burke, a thin, 19-year-old college student, has been receiving chemotherapy for leukemia, also concurrent antiemetics. She is depressed because she's had to drop out of school and now she has pushed aside her breakfast tray for the third morning in a row. When you urge her to eat, she informs you that she is not hungry and the sight and smell of the food make her sick. Two hours later, she vomits. She has no desire to eat lunch. What can you do to help Sara maintain an adequate nutritional intake?

6. John McGinnis is a retired 65-year-old janitor, who receives lower abdominal radiation for cancer of the prostate. He is a strong-willed bachelor and lives across the hall from his sister Mary in a large apartment building. Mary fixes John's meals, but because she has a job, she's unable to accompany him to the hospital for his treatments. John, who has always worried about regularity, eats bran cereal for breakfast and occasionally takes "a little phos-soda." Is there any reason he shouldn't?

7. Frank Calder, a 65-year-old retired postmaster with dentures, has developed severe stomatitis as a result of methotrexate therapy. When you examine his mouth, you see red, swollen mucosa and ulcerations on his palate. Mr. Calder complains that the lesions are extremely painful and he has much difficulty expectorating. You notice that he seems very weak. How can you make him more comfortable?

8. Betsy Seeger, a perky 8-year-old with long brown hair, is receiving prophylactic whole brain radiation for leukemia. She is popular in school and enjoys playing with her friends, but you know this could change and present problems for her when she loses her hair. You want Betsy to be happy and continue her normal activities. What suggestions can you make?

(Answers on page 177)

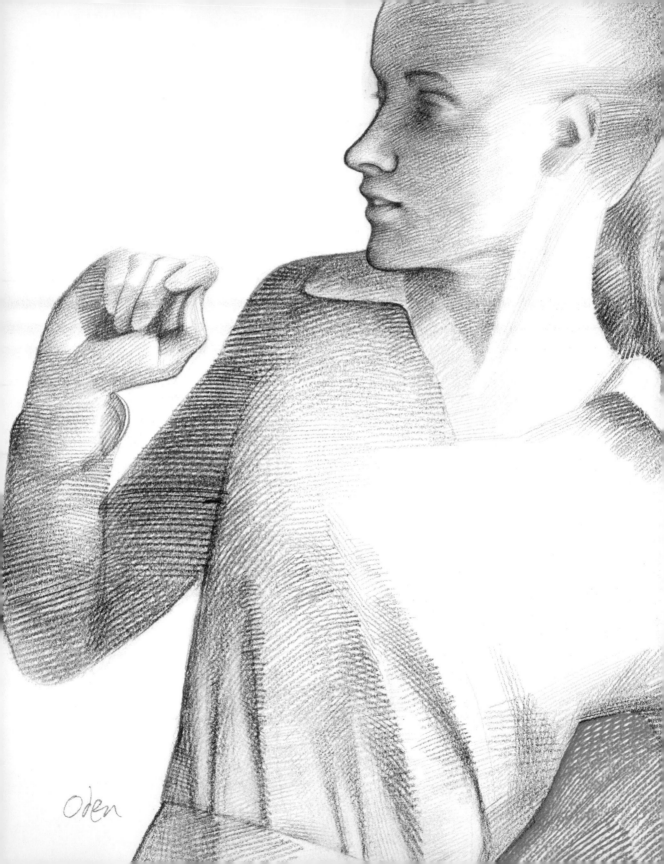

CARING FOR PATIENTS WITH CANCER OF THE THORAX

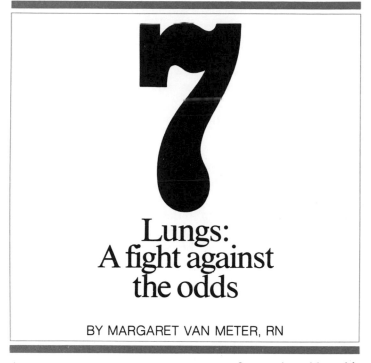

Lungs:
A fight against
the odds

BY MARGARET VAN METER, RN

A PATIENT WITH CANCER OF THE LUNG faces grim odds — his chances of surviving five years after treatment hover around 10%. If you aren't careful, knowing that fact can disrupt your nursing care.

Not that you would ignore the patient. But knowing his prognosis, you might let your sympathy interfere with your nursing judgment. I've heard nurses say, "He'll probably die soon anyhow. Why not make him as comfortable as possible now? Why not spare him the agony of postop exercises and coughing?"

But let's look at it another way: Why not do everything you can to make the rest of his life — months and possibly years — as happy and full as possible? The best way to do that is to give him your most efficient, knowledgeable care after surgery. George's story is a case in point.

"Hanging on and getting worse"
Two years ago, George R., a 43-year-old machinist went to his doctor complaining of progressive dyspnea and "fullness" in his chest, fatigue, night sweats, anorexia, and a persistent, hacking cough that produced thick sputum, particularly in the

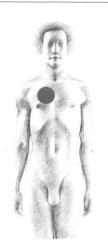

Pathophysiology:
What you should know
Lung carcinoma starts in the bronchial epithelium, more frequently in the right than the left lung. The lesion, which may be hard and nodular or soft and friable, usually develops from the epithelium of the primary and segmental bronchi; less frequently from the peripheral bronchi.

The primary lesion may project into the bronchial lumen or spread with limited intrabronchial extension into surrounding normal tissue. Eventually, through local extension, the tumor transgresses the pleural plane and extends into large and small blood vessels. It may also extend medially into the trachea, either directly or by lymph node metastases.

The primary tumor may remain small or it may spread to the other lung. And the lungs are frequently a secondary site for cancers in other areas of the body. Although lung cancer can metastasize to any organ, six sites predominate: the regional lymph nodes, the liver, the bones — especially the vertebrae, the ribs, and the sternum, the adrenal glands, and the kidneys.

morning. Although these symptoms are common to several minor respiratory diseases as well as lung cancer, George's doctor was suspicious. He knew that George had been smoking 2½ to 3 packs of cigarettes a day for well over 20 years. And George claimed that his symptoms had been "hanging on and getting worse" for three months — a hallmark of lung cancer.

One symptom that George didn't have was hemoptysis. Many nurses associate this with lung cancer. But it occurs in only 25% of patients with lung cancer — and only when the cancer is advanced.

George's doctor sent him to the hospital for the most common diagnostic tests: PA and lateral chest X-rays, sputum cytology and culture, and bronchoscopy. Although chest X-rays may be the first test, they aren't definitive since a lesion must measure 1 cm in diameter before it shows up on an X-ray. Other common tests include tomogram X-rays, CAT scan of the lungs, and scalene node biopsy. (Most doctors, though, reserve scalene node biopsies for patients with a palpable mass on either side of their neck.)

Patients undergoing any of these tests need a thorough explanation beforehand, since most are already apprehensive about the possibility of cancer. A sputum specimen should be taken early in the morning, when the patient's cough usually is most productive. The patient should clear his nose and throat and rinse his mouth before coughing. Then, he should cough against a closed glottis, to bring up sputum from deep in his chest.

For a bronchoscopy, the patient remains awake but sedated. Usually the doctor gives him atropine first to dry up his secretions. Then the doctor administers a local block to stifle his gag reflex and applies a topicial anesthetic to numb his throat. The doctor then spreads a slim (5 to 6 mm diameter) flexible rod down his throat and into his lungs. With miniature biopsy and visualization instruments, he looks around the lungs and takes specimens of any lesions.

After the anesthesia wears off, the patient generally has a sore throat. But when his gag reflex returns (within 2 to 3 hours) he can drink cool, soothing liquids and eat soft foods.

For George, these tests confirmed the doctor's suspicions: He had a tumor involving the middle and lower lobes of his right lung (the most commonly affected lung). He would have to undergo a thoracotomy two days later for exploration and possible resection.

The type of surgery a doctor settles on depends in part on extent of metastasis. If the patient's tumor is confined to part of one lung, the doctor will usually perform a lobectomy; if the tumor has invaded the entire lung, he'll usually perform a pneumonectomy; and if the cancer is inoperable, he'll probably simply close the chest. The surgery of choice also depends on the type of cancer cell. The major types of lung cancer fall into three categories: squamous cell, small or oat cell, and adenocarcinoma. Of these, squamous cell cancer responds best to surgery, and oat cell cancer hardly responds at all.

When I first talked to George about his impending surgery, he seemed to be taking the idea well. But I could tell he was anxious; he talked constantly and kept asking if he could have a cigarette. I tried to calm him by telling him that he had a good chance for resection. I also explained that he couldn't smoke because he needed all the respiratory reserves he could muster to undergo his surgery. In fact, to build up his strength, we would be putting him on a high-calorie, high-protein diet. Like many patients with lung cancer, George had lost lots of weight — 15 pounds in three weeks — and he was anorexic. We talked about the foods he liked and devised a list of healthful and appealing foods. I took the list to the dietitian and discussed ways to make his food more appealing (see Chapter 3).

During the two days before surgery, George was to have several tests — blood gas analysis, pulmonary function tests, and blood typing and cross-matching. The first two, I explained, were very simple breathing tests, which would show how well his lungs could stand up to surgery. Since pneumonitis and atelectasis can be complications of lung surgery, the doctor has to make sure the patient doesn't have any respiratory ailments going into surgery. The blood tests, I explained, were important because surgery to a highly vascular area, such as the lungs, usually necessitates blood "supplements" during surgery. Usually a patient undergoing lung surgery gets 500-1000 cc of whole blood or packed cells and blood components.

After George had finished his preliminary tests, I got down to what I consider the most important part of preop teaching: an explanation of chest tubes, coughing, deep breathing, exercises, and chest percussion.

A patient with a lobectomy usually returns from surgery with two chest tubes in place — one anteriorly in the second intercostal space and one laterally in the sixth intercostal space. The anterior tube draws off air from the empty pleural space, while the lateral tube draws off fluid. Together, they prevent pneumothorax and promote expansion of the remaining portion of the lung into the empty pleural space. Both tubes are connected to a water-seal drainage system.

A patient with a pneumonectomy, on the other hand, usually returns with only one chest tube, placed anteriorly in the second intercostal space (although some doctors don't insert chest tubes after a pneumonectomy at all). He needs only one tube because the goal after pneumonectomy is to allow fluids in the empty chest cavity to congeal and thus keep the mediastinum in place. Some air must remain in the empty space in the early postop period to equalize pressure between the right and left pleural cavities. But the chest tube prevents the build-up of too much, air, which could cause pneumothorax or tension pneumothorax. A chest tube in a patient with a pneumonectomy should *never* be connected to a standard water-seal drainage system (see accompanying illustration).

I always find that patients accept chest tubes more readily after surgery if they see them before surgery. As I showed them to George, I explained that, barring any complications, the doctor would probably "challenge" his lung function by clamping the chest tubes on the fourth postop day. If George could breathe comfortably with the tubes clamped and a chest X-ray showed his chest had sealed, the doctor would probably remove the chest tubes on the fifth day postop.

Finally, I talked to George about his role in postop deep breathing, coughing, chest percussion, and exercising his arms and legs.

After any type of lung surgery, I explained, a patient must deep breathe and cough periodically during the first few days to keep his lungs expanded and to remove secretions. Knowing that George would probably have a great deal of pain after surgery, I stressed the importance of his cooperating in postop exercises, coughing, deep breathing, and chest percussion. I showed him how I would help him splint his incision during coughing and deep breathing to ease the strain...and the pain. And I practiced chest percussion with him.

I also told George that he must do full range-of-motion

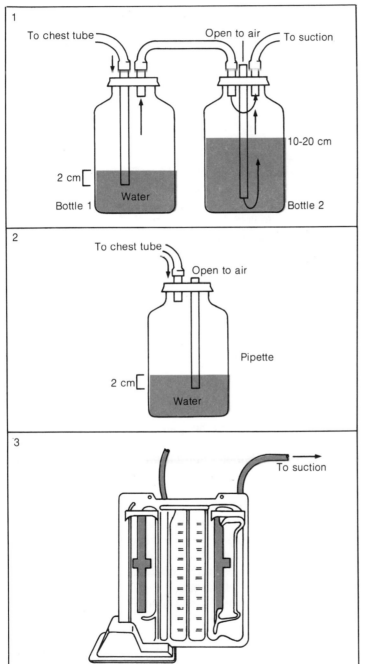

1

To chest tube
Open to air
To suction

10-20 cm

2 cm

Water

Bottle 1
Bottle 2

2

To chest tube

Open to air

Pipette

2 cm

Water

3

To suction

A liquid barrier

No matter what kind of lung surgery a patient has had, his chest tubes must be connected to a water-seal drainage system. This creates a liquid barrier between atmospheric air pressure and the negative intrapleural pressure. And that prevents the patient from sucking atmospheric air into his chest cavity.

After a lobectomy, use a standard water-seal system (Figure 1). Bottle 1 acts as a water-seal chamber and as a collection chamber for drainage. (To measure drainage, mark the liquid level on the bottle before connecting the chest tube.) Connect the chest tube to a glass pipette submerged 2 cm under water. The vent connects, via tubing, to Bottle 2 — the suction control bottle. This also has a pipette under water (the amount depends on how much suction will be applied).

After a pneumonectomy, use a special one-bottle water-seal system (Figure 2). Connect the chest tube to the vent and leave the pipette, under 2 cm of water, open to the air. *Never* connect a pneumonectomy chest tube to the under-water pipette; if pressure in the patient's chest becomes great enough, he might suck the fluid out of the bottle and into his chest.

Some doctors will order a Pleur-evac water-seal system rather than a bottle water-seal system. Figure 3 shows a Pleur-evac for a lobectomy; there is a special Pleur-evac for a pneumonectomy. With both, the principles are the same as with the bottle systems.

Getting a leg up on recovery
To protect your patient from postop emboli, start him on leg exercises soon after surgery. Holding his leg under the knee with one hand and under the heel with the other, lift it and bend it at the knee. Slowly move it toward his head. Then straighten the leg by lifting the foot upward (Figure 1). Second, holding the knee in place, pull the patient's foot toward you, then push it away from you (Figure 2). Finally, holding his leg straight, lift it about 2 inches off the bed and pull it toward you, then return it to the starting point (Figure 3). Repeat all exercises about 5 times. As the patient regains his strength, he can perform these exercises by himself.

exercises for his arms and his legs. Arm exercises (see page 82) prevent chronic shoulder stiffness caused by positioning during surgery; leg exercises (see opposite page) prevent emboli, which are a particular threat after lung surgery.

The evening before surgery, the nurse prepped George's chest. At 6:00 the next morning, I gave him his premed of Demerol, Synergan, and Atropine. Then, I accompanied him to the O.R.

Bad news, good news

In surgery, the doctor discovered a mass involving the middle lobe and part of the lower lobe of George's right lung. The left lung, fortunately, was clear. Report from pathology brought both bad news and good news: George's tumor was malignant, but at least it was squamous cell carcinoma — the cell that is most responsive to surgical therapy.

After resecting the middle and lower lobes of the right lung, the doctor closed the wound and inserted the chest tubes. Then, using a Y-connector, he attached both tubes to a single water-seal drainage bottle.

In the recovery room, the nurses added another bottle with about 10 cm of saline to act as suction control. They then attached a suction unit to the second bottle and set it at 15 cm of H_2O. This suction increases removal of fluid and air from the chest.

During the first few hours after surgery, the recovery room nurses noticed bubbles in the drainage bottle. This is normal, since the patient blows off so much excess air immediately after surgery. But bubbles don't always come from air escaping from the patient's chest; sometimes they come from a leak in the drainage system. To check the system for leaks, the nurses clamped the tubes close to George's chest for a few minutes. Fortunately, the bubbles stopped. If they had persisted, though, the nurses would have looked for a leak in the system and corrected it. If they hadn't, George might have developed a pneumothorax, characterized by dyspnea, cyanosis, and severe chest pain.

George's condition remained stable in recovery, so he soon returned to our unit. Over the next 24 hours, we adhered to the following routine:

• Check vital signs every 30 minutes during the first 4 hours and every 2 hours thereafter for 24 hours.

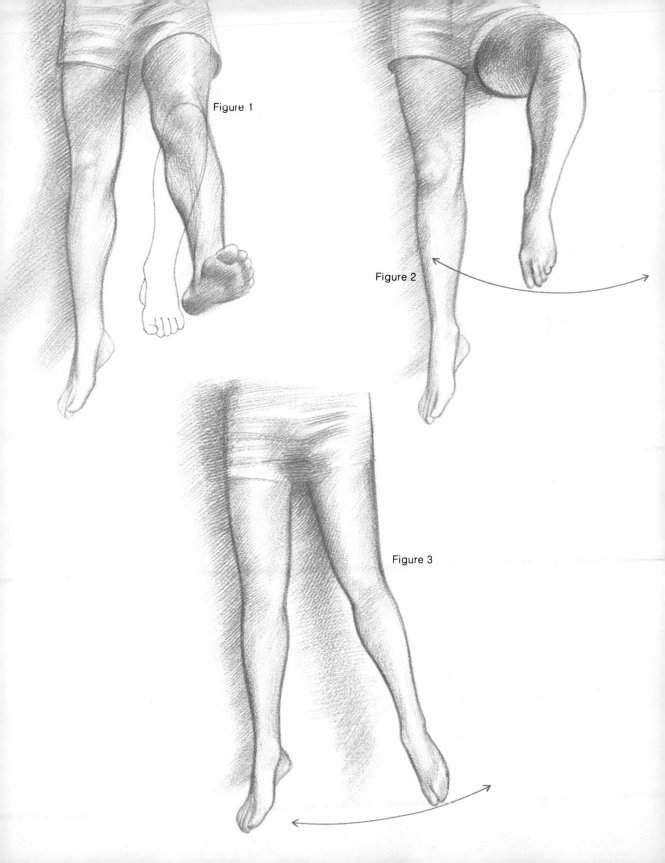

Figure 1

Figure 2

Figure 3

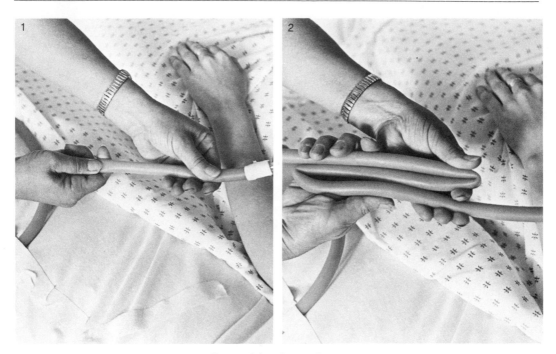

Stripping and milking the tubes
To keep chest tubes patent after a lobectomy, you'll have to strip and milk them to clear out tenacious fluids. Although mechanical strippers are available, most nurses practice the manual method. To strip a tube, pinch it hard at the proximal end with one hand and firmly tug downward on the distal end with your other hand (see photo 1). Be careful not to jiggle the tube, since that will be uncomfortable for the patient. To milk the tube, fold it together in several layers, using both hands (photo 2). Then squeeze the folded portion several times. Check the tube for proper drainage after both of these procedures.

- Record intake and output.
- Keep I.V. running at about 2500 cc per 24 hours. Too fast a flow rate increases the risk of pulmonary edema, a constant threat after thoracic surgery.
- Check secretions often for color and consistency. Initially sputum will be thick and dark with blood. But it will change to a grayish-yellow and a thinner consistency within a day. Bright red indicates hemorrhage and should be reported immediately.
- Sit the patient in a semi-Fowler's position as soon after surgery as possible (usually after an hour or two). This promotes drainage and allows air in the lower chest to rise and escape. Or, if the doctor orders, turn the patient every hour from his back to his unoperated side. Turning a patient with a lobectomy to the operated side might inhibit expansion of the resected lung.
- Check chest tubes and drainage bottle for proper functioning. During the first 24 hours, about 300 cc of drainage will collect in the bottle; initially it will be sanguineous, but it will change to serosanguineous and then to serous. Milk the drainage tube periodically. Always clamp the tubes before empty-

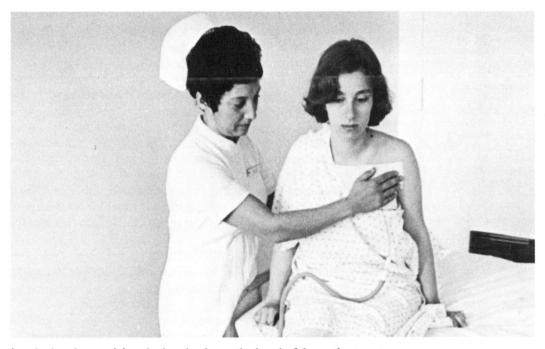

ing the bottle or raising the bottle above the level of the patient.

Throughout the early postop period, we also watched for signs of common complications: pulmonary edema, hemorrhage, atelectasis, and cardiac arrhythmias.

As soon as George arrived on our unit, we asked him to cough, deep breathe, and exercise, as I had taught him preop. Because he was still feeling the effects of the anesthesia, he cooperated with very little pain. But as the anesthesia wore off, these tasks became more painful for him — and asking him to do them became more painful for me. Still, I knew that George had to cooperate if he was to recover and try to return to a normal life. So, I gave him sedation about ½ hour before asking him to exercise and cough. I've found that many nurses withhold pain medication because they're afraid of addicting the patient. They think they're doing the patient a favor because he'll need the pain medication more if and when he enters the terminal stage. But I think withholding sedation during the painful postop period is not only cruel but also detrimental to the patient. A doctor will almost always switch a patient to a nonnarcotic oral analgesic after 5 to 7 days, so the patient hardly has time to become addicted. And if being

Cushioning the cough
During the first few days postop, have your patient cough up secretions as often as necessary. You'll have to use your best nursing judgment to decide how often is enough; remember that too much coughing can exhaust the patient.

To help the patient protect his incision during coughing, have him sit up. Stand behind him and place your hands firmly on the front and back of his chest near the incision site (see photo). Then, tell him to breathe deeply several times, inhale, and cough against a closed glottis. Or, you can cushion the cough by pressing down on his shoulder with one hand and firmly supporting the incision with your other hand.

Hormones gone haywire

Not only do lung tumors affect lung function; they also can affect other bodily functions by producing some major hormones.

• ACTH, which stimulates production of cortisol, produced most often by oat-cell carcinoma, particularly men. This produces symptoms of Cushing's syndrome (obesity, darkened skin, osteoporosis) in 50% of patients with lung cancer, and it produces hypokalemia, impaired glucose tolerance, and hypertension in even more.

• PTH, which stimulates the intestines and kidneys to increase calcium uptake, produced most often by epidermoid tumors. An excess of this hormone causes hypercalcemia, characterized by anorexia, drowsiness, nausea, constipation, and polyuria.   •

• ADH, which maintains normal levels of serum osmolality, produced most often by oat-cell tumors. This hormone can produce hyponatremia. Symptoms include lethargy, anorexia, nausea, and vomiting.

• HGH (human growth hormone), which promotes growth by stimulating protein synthesis, produced most often by large-cell and adenocarcinoma. Excess HGH causes clubbing of the fingers in 5 to 12% of patients with lung cancer and severe joint pain (much like rheumatoid arthritis) in even more.

without sedation means not coughing and deep breathing, the results can be disastrous, even fatal.

For George, the doctor had ordered Demerol 50 mg and Vistaril 25 mg every 3 to 4 hours for the first 24 hours postop. Because this kept his pain to a minimum, George cooperated fully in his postop care. By the fifth evening we had switched him to codeine by mouth.

George's secretions were rather viscous the first few times he tried to cough them up. So, we gave him a high humidity mask and stepped up our chest percussion. Fortunately, this solved the problem. If it hadn't, the doctor might have performed intratracheal suctioning or a bronchoscopy. And if that hadn't helped — if the mucus remained too thick for George to cough up — the doctor might have resorted to a tracheostomy.

A short road to recovery

Within 12 hours of surgery, George was feeling well enough to get out of bed and sit in a chair. After 24 hours, he began eating solid foods.

During the first day postop and on the third day, we ordered hemoglobin and hematocrit analyses to see if George needed a transfusion of packed cells. He didn't.

Every day, George had a chest X-ray to check for atelectasis or fluid accumulation. But the fourth day postop, the chest X-ray and his drainage indicated that his chest had sealed. He passed the "challenge" to his chest tubes with flying colors. On the fifth day postop, George was free of his chest tubes and moving more freely around the unit.

During his second week in the hospital, George started on follow-up radiation therapy. He was discharged at the end of the second week, and continued radiation therapy as an outpatient for about 6 weeks.

As of this writing, George is still alive and working part time. He has some limitations, such as heavy lifting. But generally his life is happy and unrestricted. I'll always feel that, in some measure at least, our nursing care enabled him to recover and return to a normal, productive life.

For the less fortunate

In many ways, George was lucky — lucky that he had the most "curable" type of cancer cell and that it hadn't metastasized. With early discovery and prompt surgical treatment, he has a

33% chance of surviving at least five years after surgery.

But not all patients are so lucky. Some have cancer that's more extensive or a different cell structure. For them, surgery may mean a pneumonectomy — or worse, an open-and-close thoracotomy

If your patient has had a pneumonectomy, your care will differ from the care we gave George in two important ways: turning and caring for his chest tubes.

A patient with a pneumonectomy should never be turned onto his unoperated side. That places a strain on the already-taxed remaining lung and can submerge the bronchial stump in fluid. After a pneumonectomy, turn a patient from his back to his operated side.

When caring for his chest tubes, remember your goal: to keep enough fluid and air in the pleural cavity to keep the mediastinum in place and to allow fluids to accumulate and congeal in the empty chest cavity. Since the chest tube provides an escape route only for excess air, the doctor probably will tell you to keep it clamped most of the time. Every 2 or 3 hours, though, you should release it for 15 or 30 minutes to allow excess air to escape.

Make sure, too, that the chest tube isn't connected to the underwater pipette in the drainage system. And don't connect the system to suction; it would pull the mediastinum to the operated side, creating a tension pneumothorax on the unoperated side.

Of course, a patient who's had a pneumonectomy won't drain fluid, so you won't need to milk the chest tube. And if you must apply tracheal suction for secretions, apply it very cautiously to avoid trauma to the bronchial stump.

What about a patient whose tumor has spread to both lungs, or is inoperable? Whether the doctor performs a palliative lobectomy or pneumonectomy, or simply closes the chest after exploration, your postop care will revolve mainly around giving the usual care after thoracic surgery — and lots of emotional support (see the *Nursing Skillbook* DEALING WITH DEATH AND DYING). Even if the doctor schedules the patient for radiation therapy, it will be palliative at best; it may alleviate bone pain, hemoptysis, cough, and headache (caused by brain metastasis). For an asymptomatic patient, the doctor won't order radiation therapy; its side effects would far outweigh its benefits.

Pain: A dubious distinction

About 20 years ago, cancer of the cervix was the number-one pain producer among patients with terminal cancer. But recently lung cancer has usurped that position.

Like all cancer pain, the pain of lung cancer comes not from the tumor itself but from its extension into adjacent nerves, metastasis to the bones, and pressure on adjacent organs. A Canadian study of 100 patients with lung cancer revealed six major types of pain: deep unilateral chest ache, substernal ache, severe pain in the chest wall, severe pain in the bone (particularly the lumbar spine), severe pain in the brachial plexus, and chronic, sometimes severe pain in the thoracotomy incision. The usual course of treatment begins with mild pain-killers, progressing to tranquilizers or powerful narcotics, radiation, and in extreme cases to surgery, such as cordotomy for excruciating chest wall pain.

Some doctors may try chemotherapy if the tumor is inoperable, but so far it seems to have little effect on lung tumors. Even with small or oat cell carcinoma, which seems to be most responsive to chemotherapy, the response is short-lived. The most commonly used agents include cyclophosphamide (Cytoxan), mechlorethamine (Nitrogen Mustard), methotrexate (MTX), procarbazine (Matulane), and doxorubicin hydrochloride (Adriamycin).

Of all cancer patients, those with lung cancer face the poorest prognosis. But even if they have little chance to survive five years after treatment, they probably will survive at least several months. For a dying patient, a few extra months can be a precious gift. You have to do all you can to make that time as meaningful and life-filled as possible.

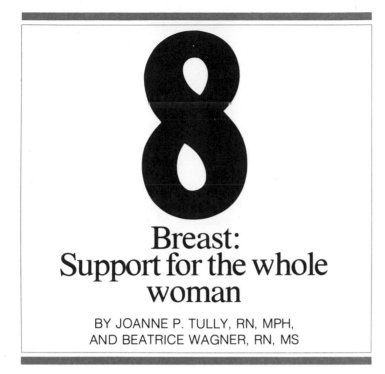

Breast:
Support for the whole
woman

BY JOANNE P. TULLY, RN, MPH,
AND BEATRICE WAGNER, RN, MS

OTHER DISEASES CAN DAMAGE a woman's body image. But, except for cancer of the reproductive organs, none strikes so near the core of her femininity or takes so much from her — physically and emotionally — as does breast cancer.

As a nurse and a woman, you can play a role in making a postmastectomy woman feel whole again. The job requires excellent physical and emotional support — but it also requires something extra. That something extra is something we believe only a woman can understand — or give. Unfortunately, patients don't always get it. Deborah is a good example.

Deborah realized the operation that took her right breast had possibly prolonged her life many years. But for her they had been empty years — or worse. She had hidden the scar from her husband for more than nine years and, she confided to us, could still hardly bear to look at it or touch it herself. She hadn't enjoyed sexual intercourse since the operation. She loved her husband and their two teenage daughters, but she said matter-of-factly, "I have nothing to live for." She hoped that someday she could join the American Cancer Society's Reach to Recovery program. But unfortunately Deborah hadn't regained her sense of wholeness; she was hardly pre-

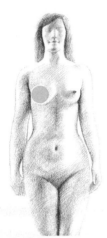

**Pathophysiology:
What you should know**
All breast carcinomas are either invasive or noninvasive adenocarcinomas that arise in the mammary epithelium. The noninvasive variety, which may become necrotic at the center, remains in the ducts. The invasive forms comprise scirrhous, medullary, and diffuse anaplastic tumors. Papillary carcinoma is the least malignant and most easily cured. Multicentric Paget's carcinoma develops within the large ducts of the nipple epithelium and erodes the nipple surface. Inflammatory carcinoma, an especially deadly form, makes the breast enlarged, indurated, discolored, and unusually warm.

Breast carcinomas usually have a single focus in one breast. Almost half of these tumors start in the upper outer quadrant and metastasize to the axillary lymph nodes. Tumors arising in the central portion (one fourth of breast carcinomas) metastasize to the mammary lymph node chain. Further growth spreads to the regional lymph nodes, neck, liver, bones, and brain.

pared to help other mastectomy patients. Sadly, Deborah died before her dream could come true.

What went wrong?
Deborah's story is sad, but positive, because it catalogues missed opportunities. If you can learn to recognize these opportunities, you won't miss them with your patients. The story begins in June, 1966, the day Deborah discovered a lump in her right breast. In September she was admitted for a biopsy and a possible mastectomy. Her preoperative X-rays were negative and all lab findings were within normal limits. In the O.R., a 3 x 4 cm lesion was removed from the superior outer quadrant of her breast. A frozen-section biopsy showed a ductal carcinoma; a radical mastectomy was performed.

The pathology report confirmed the original diagnosis and indicated that six or seven axillary nodes were positive for secondary carcinoma. No evidence of general metastasis was found. Postoperatively, Deborah received external radiation to her right axilla, the supraclavicular fascia, and the internal mammary lymphatic chain. The month after her mastectomy, her surgeon performed a prophylactic oophorectomy to prevent or slow metastasis. Afterwards she was examined by a medical oncologist three times a year for the next eight years and showed no signs of recurrent cancer.

Deborah's treatment followed the best accepted practices at that time (late 60s), but, she said, she considered her treatment close to a total failure. She felt her surgeon had failed her, because he had treated her as a breast cancer case and not as a person. When she told him about her revulsion to her scar and her complete indifference to sex after her operation, his only comment was to tell her she must have "some kind of problem with intercourse."

Deborah fared little better at the hands of her nurses. They provided competent physical care, but evidently had not assessed or intervened to help her emotional rehabilitation. She bitterly resented one of the nurses who told one of Deborah's co-workers that Deborah was a patient in the cancer clinic. Now let's see what could have been done for her.

Initiating preop teaching
As soon as your patient is admitted, familiarize her with the department and procedures, as you would any surgical pa-

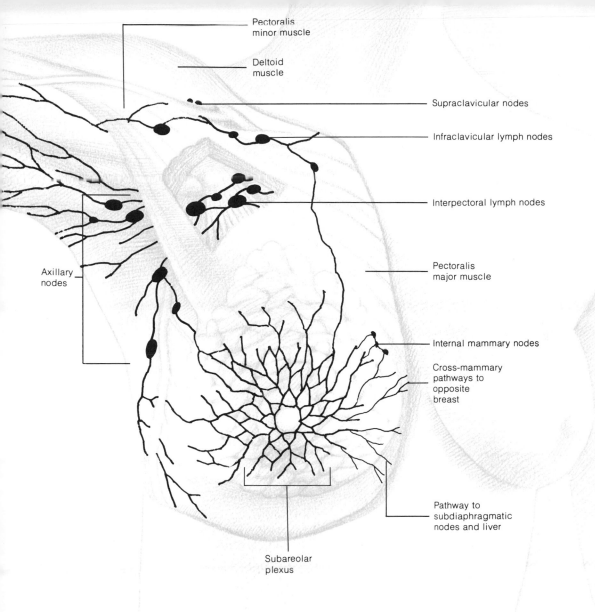

Pectoralis
minor muscle

Deltoid
muscle

Supraclavicular nodes

Infraclavicular lymph nodes

Interpectoral lymph nodes

Axillary
nodes

Pectoralis
major muscle

Internal mammary nodes

Cross-mammary
pathways to
opposite
breast

Pathway to
subdiaphragmatic
nodes and liver

Subareolar
plexus

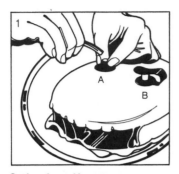

Caring for a Hemovac

1. To establish suction check all tube connections for firm seating. If evacuator isn't compressed, it may be full or may not have been activated. Remove evacuator tube from outlet "A" and place it on a sterile field. Open outlet "B," pour exudate into a basin, and replace evacuator tube to outlet "A". With evacuator on a flat surface, compress it completely and replace plug in outlet "B". This should establish effective suction and allow drainage to continue.

2. If the physician orders irrigation, fill a syringe with the proper fluid and disconnect wound tubing from tubing connector. Keep the connector sterile!

3. Insert syringe into the wound tubing and apply constant pressure until syringe is empty.

4. Replace used needle with a sterile one, refill syringe, and irrigate connector and evacuator tube so fluid runs into the evacuator. (Note amount of irrigating fluid used and subtract from total drainage.) After irrigation, empty evacuator and re-establish suction.

5. Measure amount of exudate periodically by turning evacuator on its side and reading printed calibrations. When evacuator becomes full, empty as above through outlet "B".

tient. Some patients with breast cancer are admitted for a two-stage procedure (biopsy followed by mastectomy several days later if the biopsy is positive); these patients know what they face in surgery. But many other patients with breast cancer are admitted for an excisional biopsy with a frozen section biopsy and possible mastectomy. However, before you can start preop teaching you must make absolutely sure the patient is aware that a mastectomy is possible. She will usually tell you if you ask something like, "What did doctor so-and-so tell you he was going to do for you?"

The patient is in a unique position because of the uncertainty of the mastectomy. Naturally you may be reluctant to prepare the patient psychologically for a mastectomy when you hope that it will not be necessary — and about 8 of 10 breast lumps biopsied are benign. But you must overcome this reluctance for the patient's sake. Try to individualize the teaching to your patient's specific needs, as she expresses these to you. I suggest the following steps in preop teaching:

• Find out what your patient has been told about her condition. What is planned for her and how much of the plan has been carried out?

• Describe the Hemovac and explain how it will be used to drain the serosanguineous fluid from the wound.

• Describe how the head of the bed will be raised after surgery and pillows placed under the involved arm to help drainage.

• Explain that the involved arm will feel tight after surgery and that exercises will be necessary to reduce stiffness and swelling.

• Describe the coughing exercises that will be carried out after surgery, mentioning that you (or another nurse) will help support her chest on the involved side and that coughing should come from deep in the chest rather than from the throat.

• Stress that she should remain comfortable after surgery, so she should ask for pain medication if she needs it.

• Provide emotional support by helping your patient to express her feelings and concerns about what is happening to her. Frequently, you can start the discussion by simply asking, "How do you feel about all of this?" (see Chapter 3). Try to answer all of her questions fully and help her to find answers to questions you cannot answer.

• Help the patient's family express their concerns and questions. Try to get them to understand your patient's feelings.

• Try to be with your patient when she is placed on the stretcher to go to the O.R. If possible, let her know which nurse will be with her when she returns.

After surgery, your patient may not remember all that you have told her. But preoperative teaching is vitally important, nevertheless. If your patient understands what is going on before surgery, her anxiety will be greatly reduced and she will be better able to accept her situation. Her acceptance will make her eventual rehabilitation much easier.

Try to ensure that you and others caring for her are consistent in the explanations before and after surgery. Your patient will feel confused and betrayed if she hears one answer to a particular question before surgery, and another one afterwards.

Postoperative monitoring
When your patient is returned to her room, give first priority to the usual postoperative procedures, such as checking the I.V.s, vital signs, skin color, respiratory status, level of consciousness, and the drain, if one is in place. If the patient's condition is stable in the recovery room, check her status every hour for the first 24 hours and every 4 hours for the second 24 hours. If vital signs are normal after 48 hours, you need to check them only at 8-hour periods. Watch the dressing and Hemovac for signs of excessive bleeding for 24 to 48 hours.

Position your patient on her side supported by pillows under the arm on the involved side (unless the surgeon orders otherwise). Offer your patient pain medication as ordered (usually every 3 to 4 hours) and note such medication on the chart.

Have your patient turn from side to side and flex her legs at least every 2 hours to promote circulation. If she is awake, help her with coughing and deep breathing exercises every 2 hours for 24 to 36 hours after surgery. Assist her in getting out of bed to walk briefly within 24 hours after surgery. After a few days, she should be able to walk alone.

Your patient must exercise her involved arm as soon as possible, because without exercise, the shoulder may become "frozen" in as little as 4 to 5 days. Early exercise of the involved arm will also promote lymphatic drainage and help to

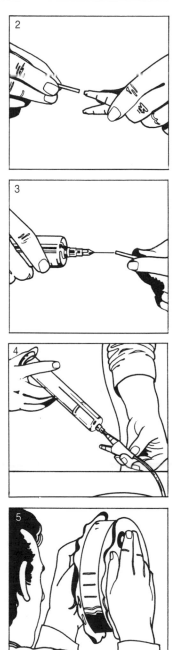

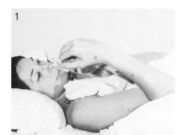

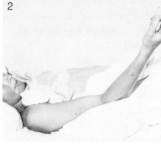

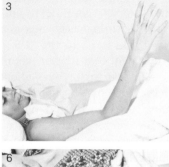

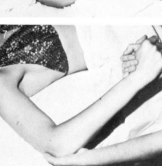

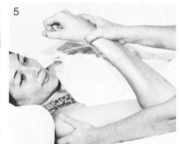

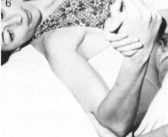

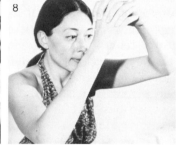

Mending the "mastectomee"

Begin active exercises immediately after surgery. Help the patient into a comfortable supine position; using a pillow, elevate her affected arm above the midline of her body. Tell her not to move her arm beyond the normal range of motion or to the point of pain. Keep track of the amount of edema in the affected arm by measuring the same part of the arm every day.

1. For elbow range of motion, instruct patient to flex and extend her elbow at least 5 times a day for a total of 5 minutes.

2. For wrist exercises, have her pronate and supinate her lower arm by turning her palm downward and then upward 5 times a day for a total of 5 minutes.

3. To exercise her hand, she should alternately clench and extend her fingers.

4. To assess brachial plexus damage, ask patient to flex and extend her elbow fully. Check her antigravity strength by asking her to hold her arm in a steady position for several seconds.

5. To check her strength against resistance, hold patient's shoulder, grasp her hand, and gently pull it toward you. Tell her to resist your pull.

6. For shoulder abduction, support patient's elbow as shown. Help her slide her elbow as far from her body as possible. Then help her bring her

upper arm across her body until it almost rests on her trunk.

7. For rotation exercises, support patient's arm as shown. Help her rotate her shoulder in direction of her head and then of her feet.

8. For active shoulder flexion exercises, patient should sit with her hands clasped in her lap. With her elbows extended at a 45° angle, she should lift her involved hand as far over her head as possible. Fully flexed, her upper arms will be close to her ears.

9. Have patient face a wall and "walk" her fingers up it until her arms are extended fully. Gradually she should move closer to the wall to increase amount of flexion.

reduce swelling. Some surgeons even have their patients lift the involved arm over their shoulder on the first day after surgery.

Many hospitals provide a formal physical rehabilitation program for mastectomy patients. If your hospital doesn't, you should see that your patient is contacted by a Reach to Recovery volunteer, who can teach the recommended exercises, or you should supervise the exercise program yourself. The Reach to Recovery manual is available from local ACS chapters.

Change the dressings as ordered by the surgeon and observe the wound carefully for early signs of infection or hematoma. Make sure that your patient eats adequately and maintains sufficient renal output.

Providing emotional support

The first days after surgery will probably be your patient's most trying, emotionally as well as physically. They will also be especially difficult days for the patient's family. If the family is at the hospital during surgery, see that they receive all pertinent information, such as when the patient is taken to the recovery room and what her general condition is. If possible, go with the family to the patient's bedside for the first post-operative visit. Later, when your patient is recovering, try to meet with the family to assess their adjustment. Are they able to accept the situation? Can they freely express their sorrow? Are the children being allowed to be a part of the family crisis, at a level comparable to their ability to understand? Are they able to meet the financial burden? If the answer is no to any of these questions, the family may need referral to the social service department.

Make sure the family understands that the postmastectomy woman now has probably the greatest need in her life to feel loved and needed. Encourage the family to frequently show how much they love and miss the patient.

One of your main jobs in nursing a mastectomy patient is to be a bridge between the family and the patient. Frequently you can get the two parties to communicate things through you that were difficult for them to say to each other.

Observe the patient closely for signs of undue stress, such as social withdrawal, excessive depression, memory lapses, or lack of appetite. Be ready to talk with your patient. Ask her to

The semantics of mastectomy

The size and location of the tumor, the extent of invasion of neighboring tissue, and the involvement of the regional lymph nodes determine the appropriate procedure for breast cancer. Generally, a surgeon performs a radical mastectomy (Figure 1, opposite page) when the tumor is large and invasive or when he finds lymph-node involvement. In this procedure he removes the entire breast, along with a significant margin of skin around the nipple, areola, and tumor, the major and minor pectoralis muscles, and the axillary lymph nodes. He also dissects the axillary vein. In the past, many surgeons performed a radical mastectomy on any woman with breast cancer. But because it involves extensive mutilation, some surgeons today use a modified mastectomy, which spares the muscles and gives the woman a more normal look.

When a surgeon finds no muscle involvement and no positive nodes, he may perform a total or simple mastectomy (Figure 2). He removes all breast tissue, but leaves muscle tissue and the axilla intact. A surgeon performs a lumpectomy or segmentectomy (Figure 3) when the tumor is small and not located near the nipple. The procedure consists of the removal of only a breast segment or tumor and 3 to 5 cm of tissue on either side of the tumor. Radiation therapy frequently follows.

describe her feelings and concerns about what is happening to her. One of the most important needs of your patient is simply to have someone to talk to. She should be allowed to grieve for her loss and to express the anger that is the natural reaction of people who must undergo the overwhelming experience of cancer surgery. Since depression and grief can recur several months after a mastectomy, encourage your patient to seek follow-up counseling. Unfortunately, no one had ever taken the time to let Deborah talk to them or referred her to any counselors.

"I've been there, too"

An ACS volunteer is invaluable in providing emotional support. Each volunteer has had a mastectomy herself, so she can say, "I know what you're going through. I went through it too and I managed." Marie, the mastectomy patient of another nurse, is a case in point. She was depressed and anxious after surgery. Her nurse counseled her and then telephoned Sue, an ACS volunteer who happened to have had a bilateral mastectomy. Sue was hard to find, but when she was finally reached by phone, she said she was playing tennis and wanted to go home and freshen up before coming to the hospital. "Never mind," the nurse told her. "This is one time when you should come as your are."

When she walked into Marie's room, Sue absolutely glowed from her workout on the court. Marie's eyes widened noticeably as she took in the trim, athletic figure in the smart tennis outfit. She had obviously expected to see some kind of physical and emotional cripple. The two chatted briefly and then Sue left. After that, Marie seemed a different woman. She was able to confront and deal with her mastectomy rationally and with confidence. If Deborah had been referred to an ACS volunteer, how different the last 10 years of her life might have been.

Postoperative teaching

Radical mastectomy operations remove the lymph nodes and lymphatic vessels draining the arm on the involved side of the body. This reduces the amount of lymphatic drainage, which ordinarily combats or controls infection due to stasis. In fact, some authorities estimate that as many as 10% of all postmastectomy women will sometime develop an infection in the

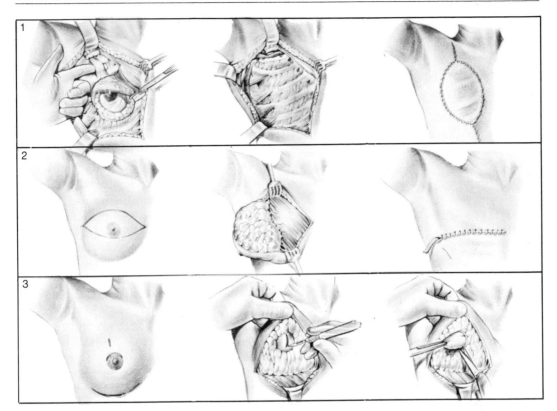

involved arm. Help your patient avoid infection and swelling by giving her the following instructions.

• Protect your affected arm by carrying your handbag or any heavy articles with your other arm. Wear your wristwatch or other jewelry on the unaffected arm.

• Never pick or cut cuticles or hangnails on your affected hand.

• Wear heavy gloves when doing light gardening.

• Use your unaffected arm when reaching into a hot oven.

• Use a thimble to avoid pinpricks when sewing.

• Apply protective insect repellent when going to areas where there may be biting insects.

• Don't permit injections, vaccinations, or blood samples to be done on your affected arm unless specifically recommended by a doctor who knows that you've had breast surgery. Be sure that blood pressure is taken on your unaffected arm.

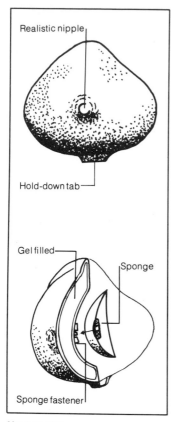

Realistic nipple

Hold-down tab

Gel filled

Sponge

Sponge fastener

Next to nature
The Second Nature breast prosthesis is one of the new "natural" prostheses being developed for mastectomy patients. It can be inserted in the cup of a bra or, with adhesive, attached directly to the skin of the chest. Many patients prefer it because it's convenient, easy to care for, and realistic in appearance. Check with the physician first before recommending it, however; he may feel that adhesive will irritate the fragile tissue of a patient who has undergone a radical mastectomy.

- Immediately wash and treat any cuts and scratches.
- Measure your arm in the same place every couple of days to detect any swelling. If your arm does swell, elevate it above your heart as much as possible and contact your doctor for antibiotic therapy.

Be sure your patient knows to tell her doctor immediately if the arm is injured in any way or if she notices any signs of infection, such as pain, redness, tenderness, or swelling.

Postmastectomy women are at a much higher risk for breast cancer (in the remaining breast) than other women. The doctor will examine your patient's breast regularly, probably monthly, but frequent breast self-examinations (BSE) are needed. Thus, you should teach your patient the proper techniques of BSE.

Selecting a prosthesis
You can help your patient adjust to her new life a great deal by helping her make a temporary prosthesis to wear around the hospital and during the first days at home. (Most surgeons won't permit their patients to be fitted with a standard prosthesis until the wound is healed and there is little chance of complications.) Putting cotton inside a premastectomy bra usually works well. At home she can sew a pocket inside the bra to hold the padding.

Advise your patient not to buy a permanent prosthesis until her doctor recommends buying one. Money spent on a prosthesis soon after surgery is wasted in many cases because the incisional site changes greatly during the first weeks following surgery. Encourage your patient to take her time buying a prosthesis and to shop around — some prostheses can cost as much as $500. Many insurance companies will pay at least part of the cost for the prosthesis if it is prescribed by her surgeon.

A large-breasted woman may require a weighted prosthesis to provide balance for proper posture. Fitted silicone-filled prostheses are usually the most natural in appearance. Brochures listing manufacturers of prostheses are available from the ACS.

A few days before your patient will be released, you should initiate discharge planning with her surgeon and any other health care professionals who will be working with the patient after she leaves the hospital, such as a Reach to Recovery volunteer. The main goal is to ensure that contact with the patient is maintained to provide continuity of care. Identify who will be checking up on the patient to see that she maintains her exercise and medication schedules. Will she need help at home with her rehabilitation or in caring for her family? Make sure someone will be available to handle such problems.

Follow-up treatment

Even when a doctor thinks that he has excised all of the cancer, he may prescribe postop treatment with radiation, chemotherapy, or hormones to ward off recurrence or metastasis. (If the cancer has metastasized widely or to the bones, he may rely on radiation or chemotherapy as the first line of treatment or as a palliative measure.)

After the trauma of breast surgery, your patient may be almost overwhelmed by the thought of additional treatment. Be sure she understands the possible side effects (see Chapters 4 and 5) but stress the expected benefits. Drugs commonly used in chemotherapy include cyclophosphamide, Adriamycin, 5-FU, and methotrexate.

For some women, the doctor may decide to follow up a mastectomy with hormone therapy. He'll elect this route only if the patient has a protein called "estrogen receptor" in her cytoplasm or carcinoma cells. If your patient will be on hormone therapy and is premenopausal, she'll receive androgens such as fluoxymesterone (Halotestin); if she's postmenopausal, she'll receive estrogens (diethylstilbestrol). Forewarn her of the possible side effects: deepening voice, facial hirsutism, and increased libido from androgen and fluoxymesterone therapy; hypercalcemia from estrogen therapy.

Unfortunately, part of hormone therapy includes additional surgery: possible adrenalectomy, oophorectomy, and hypophysectomy. Again, the thought of more surgery — particularly an oophorectomy, which further tampers with the patient's sexual identity — may be overwhelming. Support her by stressing that these measures will help retard any spread of the cancer and may prevent the need for more surgery in the future. If she's to have an adrenalectomy, explain that she'll be on permanent cortisone therapy to replace this essential hormone; if she's to have a hypophysectomy, she may need occasional steroid therapy, particularly when she's under stress. These replacement hormones will maintain her physical equilibrium. (See Chapter 11 for details on oophorectomy.)

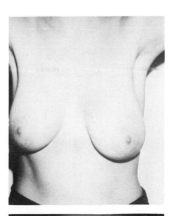

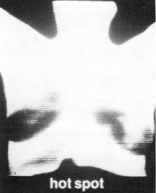

hot spot

The heat is on
Thermography shows a photographic representation of varying skin temperatures in the breast. Since inflammatory or malignant lesions have greater vascularity than normal tissue, hot spots may indicate the location of tumors. Biopsy is essential for an accurate diagnosis.

The top picture shows an enlarged left breast. A thermogram of the same patient below shows a white area or hot spot in the left breast that may be caused by a tumor.

The final failure

Unfortunately, Deborah wasn't told anything about the after-effects of a prophylactic oophorectomy. Nor did she receive any follow-up services, such as referral to Reach to Recovery. When she was last admitted in 1977, with metastatic carcinoma to bone marrow in multiple sites in her pelvis, she told me that she had never had anyone — professional or otherwise — to tell her troubles to; she had never been referred to any agency for counseling. Talking to me, she was finally able to let out much of the fear and frustration she had lived with for so long.

Deborah was never able to help other postmastectomy women directly, as she had desperately wanted to. But what she said will always be a reminder to us of the importance of the holistic approach in caring for these women. Perhaps you'll agree. In this way, at least, Deborah will get her wish.

SKILLCHECK 2

1. Rachel James is a 32-year-old clinical psychologist who had a radical mastectomy for breast cancer and has been receiving chemotherapy at a cancer clinic for nine months. She is married to a history professor and they have no children. Although metastatic lesions in her hip, pelvis, and vertebrae have partially disabled her, Mrs. James continues to work and drives herself to the clinic every week despite her husband's protests. Her major preoccupation is researching new methods for treating breast cancer, and each week she brings in more technical data. Some of the nurses find Mrs. James' attitude commendable. Do you?

2. Forty-two-year-old Evan Davis, a chain-smoking television executive, calls the physician's office one snowy morning complaining that he has another cold. He has had three colds in the past two months, all with a hacking cough. This time he reports that the cough is productive. He wants his prescription for Phenergan with codeine renewed, so his secretary can pick it up. What do you tell him?

3. Fifty-five-year-old Gayle Kaufmann is a successful food caterer. She has just had a lobectomy for cancer of the right lung, and has returned from the O.R. with anterior and lateral chest tubes. When you turn Ms. Kaufmann to her unoperated side, she suddenly complains of dyspnea and chest pain. What do you do?

4. Fifty-five-year-old Elizabeth Berkowitz had bilateral mastectomies 9 months ago. Two months ago, she developed metastases to the brain and her physician says she probably won't live much longer. She has become quite disoriented, but occasionally has lucid periods late at night when she cries out for her husband and children. Whenever Mr. Berkowitz and their two teenage sons are present, their attempts to talk to Mrs. Berkowitz fail and they wind up pacing the hall in distress. Is there anything you can do to relieve their anxiety and depression?

5. Russell Lawrence is a 66-year-old retired accountant who is four days postop from a thoracotomy for inoperable cancer of the right lung. He returned from surgery with one chest tube in place, which he immediately thought was a sign that he'd had a pneumonectomy — based on your preoperative teaching. The physician told him otherwise, and Mr. Lawrence appeared to understand. Now the chest tube is going to be removed. You are helping Mr. Lawrence out of bed when he thanks you for your preop teaching and tells you that he is relieved that the physician got all the cancer when they removed his lung. What do you do now?

6. Tillie Ritter is a spunky 78 year old, with slight arthritis of the spine, who will soon be discharged from the hospital after a simple mastectomy for breast cancer. Though large busted, she refuses to consider a temporary or permanent prosthesis for herself, claiming that they are frivolous and completely unnecessary for a woman her age. Her records and conversations reveal that she lives in an expensive retirement community, plays bridge four times a week, and participates in the social activities of several clubs. Some of the staff admire Miss Ritter's nonchalant attitude and lack of vanity. Should you be concerned?

(Answers on page 178)

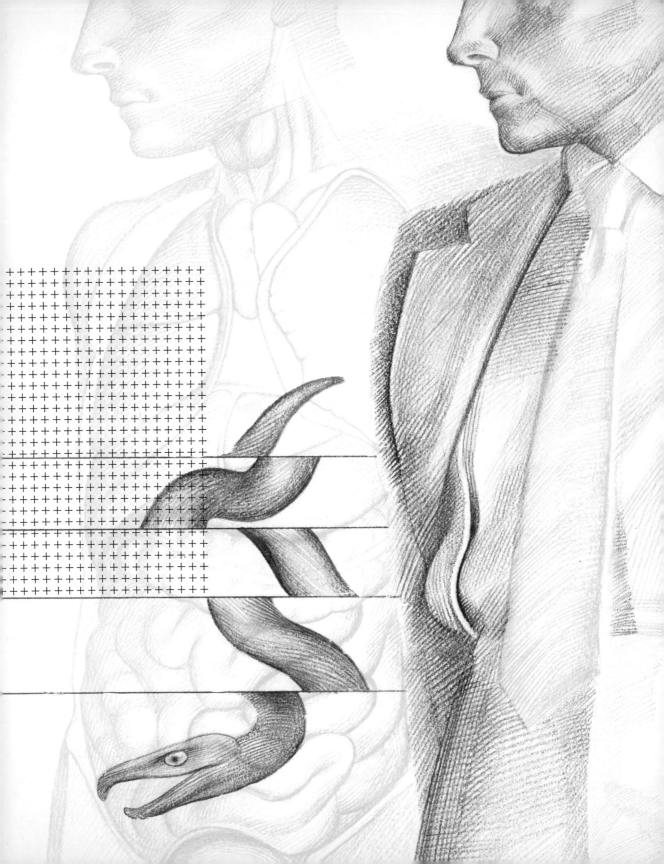

CARING FOR PATIENTS WITH CANCER OF THE ABDOMEN

Oden

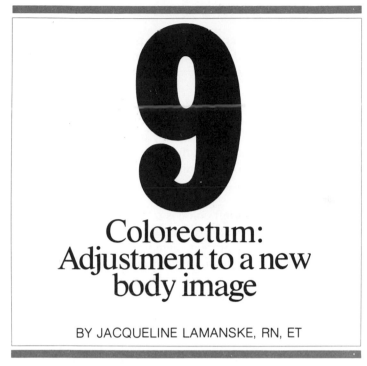

9

Colorectum: Adjustment to a new body image

BY JACQUELINE LAMANSKE, RN, ET

TO CARE FOR ANY PATIENT with colorectal cancer, you must be three people in one: the efficient nurse who gives fine in-hospital care; the compassionate nurse who gives emotional support; and the instructive nurse who teaches the patient home care. But if your patient will have a colostomy, your roles as emotional supporter and patient educator will be especially important — the patient will have to cope with the emotional trauma of his new body image and the daily care of his stoma. How can he think of surviving, let alone actually living with the dreadful duo: cancer and colostomy? Well, millions of people are living with it every day, and with more relief, ease, and comfort than your patient might think possible. With your help, he too will adjust.

Site determines surgery
Adenocarcinoma can occur anywhere in the colon or rectum, but the most common sites are the distal sigmoid and rectum. The type of surgery performed for colorectal cancer will depend on the site and extent of the tumor.

Carcinoma in the right colon is resected, with the surgeon performing a right hemicolectomy and anastomosing the ileum to the mid-transverse colon. The symptoms of cancer in this area may include mild diarrhea, abdominal discomfort, dyspepsia, weight loss and anemia, and possibly a palpable abdominal mass.

A tumor in the transverse colon may necessitate a resection including the hepatic and splenic flexures, or the surgeon may elect to do a subtotal colectomy. Before surgery, the patient may complain of a noticeable change in bowel habits, such as alternating constipation and diarrhea. Constipation may increase, and the patient may occasionally pass blood and mucus with his stool.

Cancer of the upper left colon is resected with anastomosis of the right transverse colon to the sigmoid colon. A resectable lesion in the sigmoid or rectosigmoid may call for a wide resection, with the descending colon being anastomosed to the rectum.

Relatively small tumors in the upper rectum or lower rectosigmoid may also be treated with wide resection and anastomosis. But larger lesions and those lower in the rectum will necessitate wide removal of the rectum and rectosigmoid — in other words, an abdominal-perineal resection with the construction of a permanent end-sigmoid colostomy. The doctor will suture the perineal wound closed and insert a suction catheter between the perineal floor and the skin; or he may leave the wound open with large drains, which will be removed slowly to allow healing by secondary intention. The incidence of impotency in males after an AP resection is very high. The symptoms of a cancer in this location are increasing constipation, rectal bleeding, a feeling of pressure in the rectum, and later abdominal or rectal pain.

A surgeon may perform a temporary colostomy if the lesion is totally obstructive and the surgeon feels that effective preoperative bowel cleansing is impossible. Some patients will receive preoperative irradiation to the site of a large rectal lesion in hopes of reducing its size. And some patients will receive postoperative chemotherapy after a recuperative period following their surgery.

Since colorectal cancer occurs most often in the distal sigmoid and rectum, many cancer patients face the prospect of living with a colostomy. This chapter focuses on their care. But if your patient can be treated with a partial colectomy and anastomosis of the colon — you should give the same sym-

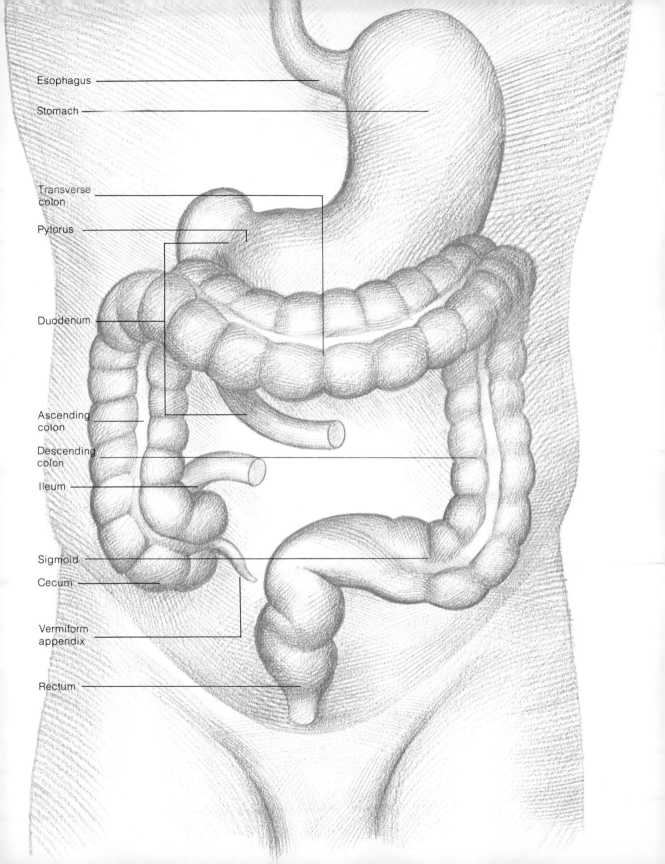

Esophagus

Stomach

Transverse
colon

Pylorus

Duodenum

Ascending
colon

Descending
colon

Ileum

Sigmoid

Cecum

Vermiform
appendix

Rectum

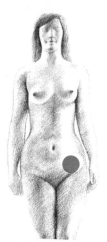

**Pathophysiology:
What you should know**
Benign polyps, longstanding ulcerative colitis, and familial polyposis all prefigure colorectal cancer. Cancer of the colon tends to grow slowly and remain localized for a long time. Three-quarters of the primary lesions originate in the sigmoid colon. Large bowel tumors are usually adenocarcinomas that appear either as friable, easily bleeding polypoid lesions, or as hard-edged craters that obstruct the lumen of the bowel. Obstruction leads to the typical pattern of alternating diarrhea and constipation which is the curse of so many patients.

Colorectal cancer may spread by direct extension into the bowel wall and adjacent tissues or by metastasis through the blood and lymph system to the regional lymph nodes, the liver, and in advanced stages, the lungs.

pathetic emotional support and immediate postop care of the incision.

Early teaching for better adjustment
Preoperative teaching is as crucial to your patient's well-being and later adjustment as any nursing procedure. In fact, your attitude toward the colostomy will in subtle ways convey itself to your patient, and greatly influence his attitude. You should include the family as well as the patient in your explanations and teaching. Find out what the patient knows of the surgery he's about to have, then reinforce his understanding and correct any misapprehensions. I always have a simple chart on hand to familiarize the patient with his GI tract. And I use another anatomy chart to show the postsurgical GI tract — not so much to dwell on what will be removed as to reassure the patient about how much really remains. He may not know, for example, that digestion and nutritional absorption don't really require a colon because they take place in the small intestine anyway.

Be prepared to discuss the stoma with him in detail. He ought to know what it is, that its natural color is red, and that right after surgery it will be rather swollen but will decrease in size in a few weeks. I also give informational booklets discussing life with a colostomy both to the patient and to his family.

When the patient has begun to absorb this much, you can show him the sort of appliance he will wear. People who have heard the word "bag" usually find this conception upsetting. One gentleman was going to refuse his surgery because all he could picture was wearing a garbage bag. When he saw the slim appliance he would actually use, he was greatly relieved. I proceeded to explain how it gets attached to the skin, that it is virtually odor-proof, and that it can't be detected under even tight clothing; he was reassured.

After explaining the stoma, try to arrange a preop visit by a recovered ostomate. That way, the patient will see someone else who has undergone the surgery he's about to have and who has obviously emerged healthy and productive.

Before surgery, check the site for the stoma. Its location is extremely important. A colostomy will emerge through the rectus muscle, usually on the left abdomen below the beltline. It must be located away from the umbilicus, from bony prominences, and from areas of scarring. It should be on a relatively flat surface for the fixing of an appliance, and it should be free of creases and dips when the patient sits, stands, bends, squats, or stoops. And it has to be in a place that he can easily see. Only if these conditions can be met will the patient be free of appliance leakage, skin breakdown, and the emotional upheaval these problems can bring.

Sometime during adaptation to his colostomy, the patient should be seen by an enterostomal therapist if available. An ET is an RN specially trained and certified in the care and rehabilitation of patients with all types of abdominal stomas. The United Ostomy Association has a list of pamphlets, booklets, slides, and other helpful articles prepared by ostomates, ETs, and other professionals that will be extremely useful to you and your patient.

Usually you should begin bowel preparation for surgery two days preoperatively. This generally includes a clear liquid diet and a nutritional supplement, a stool softener, vitamins, a phosphasoda, colonic irrigations, and neomycin and erythromycin base therapy beginning the afternoon before surgery. If the patient is in a poor nutritional state because of chronic debilitative disease or has received cobalt therapy, you may have to give him parenteral hyperalimentation preoperatively. Take daily weights before and after surgery. Before surgery, you also should instruct the patient in inhalation therapy. If possible, show him the recovery room and the intensive care unit and introduce him to personnel there.

Attention to tubes and lines

After surgery, the patient will have a peripheral I.V., a CVP line, a Foley catheter attached to bedside drainage, and an NG tube or a gastrostomy tube (or bowel splint), which will be attached to suction or gravity drainage. Your care routine may be as follows:

• Keep the peripheral I.V. open in case you have to give blood, fluids, or medications.

• For the subclavian CVP line, use the best no-touch sterile technique when changing dressings. Cleanse a 3 cm radius around the tube with 95% alcohol. Then, apply tincture of benzoin, followed by tincture of Betadine and Betadine ointment. Finally, cover the insertion site with sterile 2x2s and occlusive dressing.

• Record intake and urine output hourly; then, resume an

every-eight-hours routine. Every day, clean the meatus with zephiran solution followed by Betadine ointment. Anchor the Foley catheter securely to the patient.

• Cleanse the incision daily with hydrogen peroxide and change dressing p.r.n. Cleanse the site of the gastrostomy tube daily with peroxide; apply Betadine ointment and cover with a sterile 4x4. Anchor the tube with tape.

• Give IPPB treatments and continue them for five days. Turn the patient and have him deep breathe and cough regularly while he remains on bedrest. The evening of surgery, have him dangle his feet over the side of the bed, then, increase activity as tolerated the morning after surgery.

If your patient has a nasogastric tube, it probably will remain in place for several days postop; if he has a gastrostomy tube, it may remain in place as long as 14 to 21 days. With either tube, be sure to give good mouth care and use glycerine swabs (see Chapter 10). Before removing either tube, make sure gastric drainage isn't excessive, peristalsis is normal, and the abdomen isn't distended with gas. For instructions on removing an NG tube, see Chapter 10. Before removing a gastrostomy tube, clamp it for 24 hours to make sure he can tolerate it. If the patient doesn't experience nausea and the residual from the tube is under 50 cc, start him on clear liquids. If he tolerates this diet for 24 hours with no nausea and low residual from the tube, he can proceed to full liquids. From there, he can rapidly progress to a normal diet. By now, the CVP line will have been removed.

Complications of major colon surgery include bleeding, wound infection, abscess formation, fistula, wound dehiscence, anastomotic leakage, mechanical obstruction, urinary tract infection, thrombophlebitis, pulmonary emboli, and pneumonia. Particularly in the early postop period, watch for warning signals: elevation in TPR, change in blood pressure, abdominal distention, nausea, vomiting, changes in output (both gastric or urinary), gross bleeding, or change in mental status.

Fit, stick, and apply
Immediately after surgery, an appliance may be applied over the stoma, even though no stool is expected for a few days. The appliance will collect any serosanguineous drainage and will keep the parastomal skin dry and protected. The appliance

should be transparent so the doctor can check the color of the new stoma without having to disturb the seal. Because the first stools will be soft, they will be irritating to the skin. So, the patient may need a skin protector.

When changing the appliance you'll need:
• an open-end drainable colostomy appliance
• rubber bands or closure clamp, unless the appliance has this attached
• skin protectors such as karaya rings or Stomahesive, unless the appliance already has karaya attached to the back
• small scissors
• measuring guide
• gauze squares

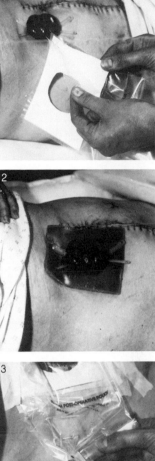

To fit the appliance, measure the stoma and cut the appropriate size opening in the pouch, allowing ⅛" clearance all around (photo 1). With warm water, gently clean the parastomal skin and dry it *thoroughly*. Place fresh gauze squares on the stoma to keep drainage from the cleansed skin.

Slightly moisten a karaya ring and rub in the moisture until the ring turns sticky. Place the ring close around the stoma and press gently so it adheres to the skin. No skin should show between the base of the stoma and the inner edges of the ring (photo 2).

Peel the paper backing off the appliance. Then apply the appliance over the stoma so its adhesive area sticks to the karaya ring, with the opening centered evenly around the stoma. Gently press around the stoma so that the adhesive bonds to the karaya ring and the surrounding skin. Press any wrinkles out carefully; wrinkles only make tunnels through which the fecal output will leak onto the surrounding skin.

If you use Stomahesive in place of the karaya washers, cut the opening to fit the stoma much as you've cut out one for the bag; only this time, make it a perfect fit without any margin of exposed skin. Then attach the shiny side of the Stomahesive to the appliance; peel off the paper backing on the other side and apply the appliance to the skin.

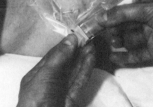

Now close the bottom of the pouch by folding it upward twice, then fanfolding (photo 3). Fasten it with a rubber band or clamp to prevent leakage out of the bottom.

If everything is in order and the seal directly around the stoma is watertight, the appliance will stay fastened securely in place for at least 24 hours. It can stay longer if the seal remains intact. In fact, with Stomahesive, some users have gotten 5 to 7 days out of one appliance.

At the first sign that the output is about to leak out beneath the seal, change the appliance. Don't wait for actual leakage. Not only will it irritate the skin; it also will upset the patients.

Empty the appliance when it's about one-third full; if it gets too full, it will pull away from the skin. And if you've planned it properly, it will be much easier to empty into a measuring container, which you must do as long as the patient is unable to go to the bathroom. For the early postop patient, the best position for the pouch is diagonal, with the end falling slightly over the hip. As the patient turns from side to side, the output can still flow to the bottom of the pouch.

Later, when the patient is up and about and can empty his own appliance while sitting on the toilet, it should be placed so that the bottom of the pouch points toward his feet.

The patient with a transverse colostomy will always need a skin barrier that fits snugly around the stoma, and should always wear an odorproof open-end appliance.

With a sigmoid colostomy, though, the stools eventually will become formed and less irritating to the skin. At that stage, he won't need a skin barrier any more. The opening in a small adhesive-backed appliance should be cut about ½" away from the stoma to allow formed stool to pass through. If the opening is cut too close, the formed stool will undermine the appliance and lift the whole thing away from the body. Later, the patient can use a closed-end appliance when his bowel evacuation becomes regulated. He shouldn't use a closed-end appliance if it needs to be changed more than once in 24 hours. In that case, an open end appliance that may be emptied would be better.

Gaining bowel control

Chances are, a patient with a sigmoid colostomy will eventually develop bowel control through periodic irrigations of his stoma. Some patients may not benefit from the routine stoma irrigation: a patient who had an erratic, irritable type bowel prior to surgery; a very elderly patient; one with poor eyesight or limited use of his hands; a patient with a temporary colostomy (because the bowel is expected to be rejoined in a relatively short time); a patient with a transverse colostomy; and a patient who is terminally ill.

The irrigation takes about an hour from start to finish, although not all of this time need be spent in the bathroom. It involves instilling about 1 quart of lukewarm water hung at shoulder level, inserting a catheter or preferably the tip of a cone into the stoma, then letting the water run from the container into the colon. Because there is no sphincter to retain the water, the cone tip plugs the stoma so that the water cannot be expelled prematurely. (If using a catheter, a shield of some kind should be used to serve this purpose — for instance, a soft baby nipple can be used by inserting the catheter in the wide end of the nipple and through the nipple so that the catheter protrudes a few inches beyond.) As the water flows against the walls of the colon, it builds up pressure and stimulates muscle contractions that evacuate the bowel.

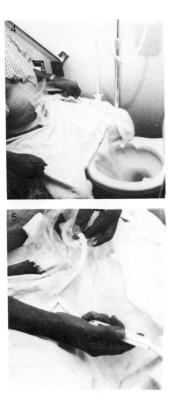

If done routinely at about the same time every day or every other day, irrigation will empty the bowel and prevent stoma activity between irrigations. How long the bowel takes to get used to emptying at a regular time will vary from patient to patient.

Before irrigating, assemble your equipment: irrigation bag with tubing and cone (or catheter), irrigation sleeve and belt, and clips (or rubber band). Fill the bag, and hang it so the bottom is at shoulder level. Place a chair facing the toilet and have the patient sit on this. After his rectum heals, he may sit on the toilet.

Remove the used pouch and replace it with a plastic irrigating sleeve — place the bottom of the sleeve in toilet bowl (photo 4). Lubricate the end of the cone (or catheter). Then briefly release the clamp on the tubing so water runs through and empties air out of tubing. Close the clamp again.

Gently insert the tip of the cone into the stoma and hold it firmly against the stoma (photo 5). Control the clamp so water flows in slowly. (If stool appears around the cone while you're introducing water, shut off the clamp, remove the cone, allow the stool to pass, and then continue with irrigation. If water doesn't appear to be going in, try gently changing position of the cone until water begins to flow.)

After water is instilled, clamp the tubing and remove the cone. Close the top of the sleeve with clips. Most of the water and some stool will empty within 15 to 20 minutes; then you can rinse the sleeve by running water through it. Fold the bottom up even with the top, fold over twice and clip. The patient can then go rest in bed or bathe and shave. An hour after you began instilling the water, you can remove the sleeve and reapply a pouch. Empty the sleeve, rinse it with a mild soap solution and cool water, then hang it up to dry. Keep all irrigating equipment together at the patient's bedside, so it doesn't get misplaced, and it will then be ready to use next time. When irrigating a patient who's in bed, hang the water bag from an I.V. pole, making sure that the bottom of the bag is low enough. After putting the sleeve on, fold up the bottom of it, fanfold it, close it with a strong rubber band, and let it rest on the bed rest between the patient's legs. Then continue with the irrigation.

Teach — but take it slowly

In the immediate postop period, the patient's main concern is his discomfort. But as he recovers from surgery, he'll have to learn how to take care of his stoma at home. You must make him as comfortable as you can and take care of his basic physiologic needs before he can be receptive to learning anything.

At the onset of recovery you can start passive teaching by explaining stoma care as you perform it. While you are doing each step, explain it aloud and give the reason. Then, when the patient is alert and feeling better, he'll be somewhat familiar with the process and can begin to learn it in depth.

Try to gradually incorporate the patient's assistance into his care. This builds his confidence. A good first step is having him learn how to manage the closure clamp. Next you can try letting him empty the appliance while sitting on the toilet. Third, you can let him help with skin care and fastening the appliance on himself.

If the first few attempts don't work, remind the patient that it took a few times of trying to learn to ride a bicycle, or to cook the roast without burning it, and much more effort to learn to drive. Encourage him; praise and success build confidence.

Before he leaves the hospital, he should be doing his own care with your psychological support. If an enterostomal therapist is available, he should certainly have seen one. Now's a good time, too, for another visit from a fellow ostomate.

He should be introduced to different appliances. Many patients keep using one appliance whether they have trouble with it or not, simply because they know of no others. Your patient should be discharged from the hospital with at least a 3-4 week supply of equipment, and he should know where he can buy it in his community. If he's indigent, the Social Service Department should advise him on obtaining supplies.

Relating to others

Naturally a patient with a new colostomy worries about the odor. Reassure him that, with routine stoma irrigations or an odorproof appliance and an appliance deodorant, the appliance will be virtually odor-free. He should apply the liquid deodorant to a cotton ball or piece of tissue and put it in the bottom of the pouch through the emptying spout.

Expelling gas through the stoma can cause a gurgling sound. But if the patient folds his arms and gently presses against the stoma, it will be effectively muffled. Once in the pouch, the gas can't escape on its own, so the wearer will later have to open the bottom and press the appliance against his abdomen to dispel it. All patients will have a certain amount of gas, though some foods produce more of it than others. These include beans, onions, cabbage, and carbonated drinks. The patient may wish to avoid these foods at social times, or eat less of them than usual, to control this effect.

A new ostomate may also think that he'll have to buy special clothes to hide the unsightly bulge of the appliance or stoma. Reassure him that he'll be able to wear his normal wardrobe and that the appliance will be undetectable — even under a bathing suit.

Both sexes, after colostomy, will wonder about their sexual function and their altered body image. If a marriage was happy before surgery, it will usually remain so after surgery.

The female patient may note some discomfort with intercourse until the perineal wound has healed. But the patient and the mate should know that the stoma will not be injured by contact during these intimate moments.

Men will seldom have trouble with impotency following tumor resection and anastamosis of the colon. But men with wider resection performed for cancer of the rectum and those left with colostomies almost always will be impotent. (See Chapter 12 for a discussion of the psychological problems impotence can create.)

Excellent pamphlets on the topic of sex and the ostomate

are available from the United Ostomy Association or the American Cancer Society. These are full of information for males and females, married or single.

Once the immediate postoperative period is over, the patient can resume his normal activities. Teachers can return to their classroom, students go back to school, nurses go back to work, firemen go back to climbing ladders and fighting fires, and housewives and mothers go back to being able to take care of their homes and families again.

In the community
No patient should leave the hospital without knowing that there's more help available to him after he leaves nursing care. A visiting nurse should call on the patient after his return home to be sure he's able to cope. Attendance at ostomy meetings after discharge will keep him informed about new appliances and techniques. If there's no local ostomy chapter in the area, tell him about the United Ostomy Association. It will gladly send him information about the organization and let him know the location of the nearest group. And he should know about an enterostomal therapist in his area. If he lives too far for you to know who it is, the United Ostomy Association can give him that professional's name too. Write United Ostomy Association, 1111 Wilshire Boulevard, Los Angeles, California 90017, phone (213) 481-2811.

Can the ostomy patient accept surgery and learn to live a healthy, productive life? The answer is yes. Gone, surely, are the days when patients were left on their own to cope with stoma care by trial and error. By adequate patient preparation and good postoperative care and teaching, and by acquainting the patient with the professional services that are available to him after he leaves the hospital, you can help him meet this challenge and make a complete adjustment to it.

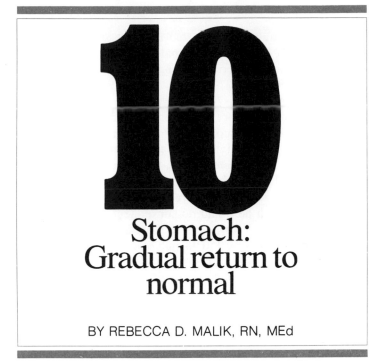

Stomach:
Gradual return to
normal

BY REBECCA D. MALIK, RN, MEd

SURGERY OFFERS THE ONLY way to cure stomach cancer, so nursing care revolves around that treatment. To give optimum care, you should know the types of gastrectomies most frequently performed (and how a radical subtotal gastrectomy differs from a total gastrectomy), the preoperative and postoperative nursing duties (including how to manage a patient with nasogastric tubes and how to help him progress to a normal diet), and possible complications (such as the "dumping syndrome" and how to control it).

Indigestion: The first warning

Stomach cancer can be cured if it's diagnosed and treated early enough. But that's not always possible. The first symptoms — vague indigestion and slight loss of appetite — appear so gradually the patient usually isn't aware of them.

Later, more obvious symptoms develop: nausea, vomiting, abdominal distention with flatulence, and gross anorexia with actual food repugnance. The patient may complain of not feeling well — of feeling that "something is wrong."

As the disease progresses, he may experience pain similar to that of a peptic ulcer. A stomach mass usually can't be pal-

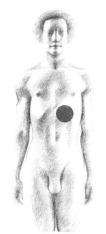

**Pathophysiology:
What you should know**
Most stomach cancers occur in the pyloric segment and near the lesser curvature. Differentiating cancer of the stomach from benign tumors, large polyps, and chronic ulcers, can be difficult for many of the symptoms are the same: loss of weight and appetite, anemia, and fatigue. In fact, these benign conditions can be precursors of cancer.

Carcinoma of the stomach infiltrates rapidly, spreading to the regional lymph nodes, omentum, liver, and lungs by the following routes: the walls of the stomach, duodenum, and esophagus, the lymphatic system, adjacent organs, the bloodstream, the peritoneal cavity, transplantation, and transluminal implantation.

pated, though, unless it's located near the pylorus. At this stage, the patient will appear pale because of secondary anemia, and he'll experience progressive weight loss and progressive weakness.

A typical patient was Mr. M., age 54, who had lost 30 pounds in 4 months before being hospitalized. He complained of vague abdominal discomfort, malaise, and general weakness that had progressively increased over the previous 6 months. Two years earlier, Mr. M. had experienced frequent episodes of localized midabdominal pain. After a routine physical examination, he'd been prescribed antacids for a few weeks, after which he'd had no subsequent pain.

Upon admission, Mr. M.'s temperature was 98.8° F. (37.1°C.), blood pressure 150/96, pulse 86, and respirations 20. He was pale, tense, and cachectic, but had no signs of jaundice or clubbing. His liver span was 10 cm by percussion, and the liver edge was palpable below the costal margin, indicating enlargement. Mr. M. had some vague tenderness in his epigastrium, but no palpable masses. The rest of his physical examination findings were normal.

Because the doctor suspected stomach cancer, he ordered certain blood chemistry studies for Mr. M. The results were: hemoglobin, 11 Gm/100 ml (normal is 14 to 18 Gm/100 ml); hematocrit, 32% (normal is 40% to 54%); stained red cell examination, microcytosis (cells are smaller than normal), and hypochromia (cells have less than normal color). All these results indicate anemia.

Mr. M. also underwent the usual diagnostic studies for stomach cancer. His upper GI series — a radiological examination with barium swallow — showed a filling defect and a distortion of the mucosal pattern in the antral region. Gastroscopy (done with a fiberoptic endoscope) revealed a massive lesion in the region of the fundus with a very shallow ulceration in the middle and nodular border. Since all of these findings are consistent with the suspected diagnosis — malignant lesion of the ulcerative variety — several biopsies were taken. (Alternately, a brush cytology is sometimes done, in which specimens of the stomach lining are obtained by brushes.) The studies all confirmed cancer.

A chest X-ray, scans of the liver and pancreas, and other laboratory tests showed no evidence of any metastasis to the lungs, liver, pancreas, or other surrounding organs. After a surgical consultation, Mr. M. was scheduled for a radical subtotal gastrectomy.

Before surgery: Giving honest answers

The treatment of choice for stomach cancer is a radical subtotal (partial) gastrectomy. This procedure involves resecting the tumor and surrounding area, then connecting the remainder of the stomach to the duodenum (Billroth I procedure) or to a loop of the jejunum (Billroth II procedures). The Billroth II, which has several variations, is done most frequently (see page 110).

Since all these procedures involve removing one-half to two-thirds of the stomach, the patient's greatest concern usually is how he'll be able to live without his stomach. For example, he'll want to know how he'll eat; whether he'll be able to eat regular food, or be restricted to a special diet for the rest of his life.

So, perhaps the most important thing you can do for your patient preoperatively is reassure him that he will be able to eat regular foods (within certain guidelines) and that he will be able to lead a normal life.

But if your patient is having a total gastrectomy, the picture is somewhat bleaker. Total gastrectomy involves removing the entire stomach and surrounding area including the regional lymph nodes, with anastomosis between the ends of the esophagus and the jejunum. Although chances of the cancer recurring are much less with a total gastrectomy than with a subtotal gastrectomy, chances of postoperative complications are much greater. Recovery is slower, and resumption of a normal diet takes longer.

Begin your preop teaching just as soon as possible. Most patients are admitted to the hospital 2 to 3 days before surgery, so you'll have plenty of opportunities for teaching. Include the patient's family in your teaching sessions whenever possible, so they'll know what to look for and how to help the patient postoperatively.

In discussing what to expect after surgery, emphasize that the patient will need to change his position every 2 hours. This will make him more comfortable and help prevent pulmonary and vascular complications. Stress the importance of taking deep breaths and coughing every 1 to 2 hours and of trying to move about when ordered. This will help prevent complications and promote respiration.

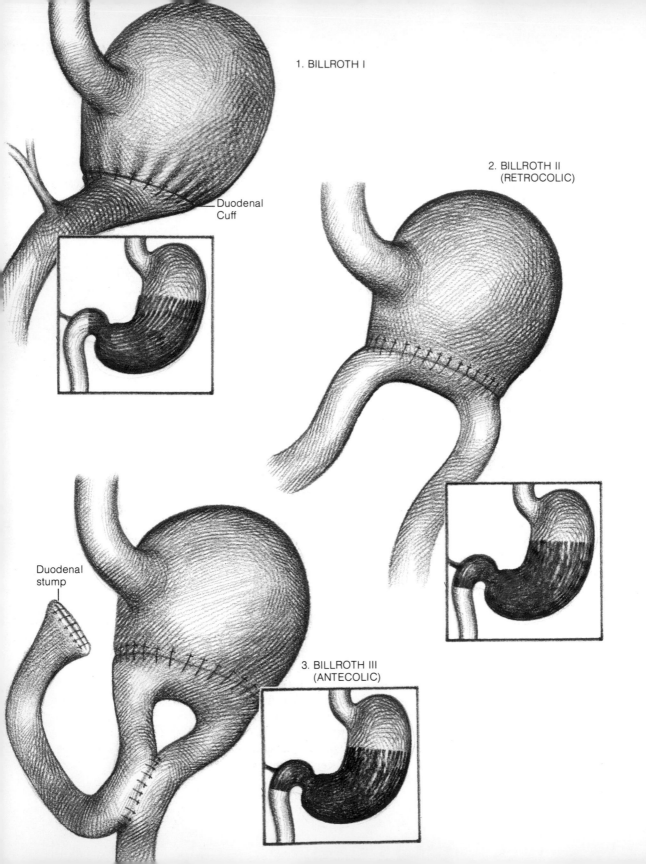

1. BILLROTH I

Duodenal Cuff

2. BILLROTH II (RETROCOLIC)

Duodenal stump

3. BILLROTH III (ANTECOLIC)

Be sure to prepare him for the tubes he'll have postoperatively — a nasogastric tube connected to suction and, if he has a total gastrectomy, chest drainage tubes. Explain that he'll be fed intravenously until peristalsis resumes, and that he can tolerate oral feedings.

If he's physically debilitated before surgery, he may need certain preoperative measures to strengthen him. Such measures might include a nutritious nonresidue diet, supplemental vitamins B and C, intravenous infusions of 5% glucose in saline solution to correct fluid and electrolyte imbalance, and blood transfusions to combat anemia.

After surgery: Tube precautions

Your preop teaching efforts will pay off postoperatively if you've established a trustworthy relationship with your patient. Be sure to review and reinforce your preop instructions about changing positions, deep-breathing, and coughing. Since the patient will have a high abdominal incision, this will be painful. Give him pain medications as ordered. If he does these exercises effectively, he may not need intermittent positive pressure breathing treatments.

Your patient won't be allowed anything by mouth for several days, because he'll have a nasogastric (NG) tube connected to suction. Drainage from this tube may contain blood for the first 12 hours after surgery. If the blood is excessive, or if any blood appears after that time, be sure to report it to the doctor.

You'll need to check the patency of the NG tube frequently, but irrigate it only as ordered by the doctor. Since the surgeon placed the tube during the gastrectomy to protect the suture line, don't try to move or remove it. This could cause abdominal distention. If the tube stops functioning, notify the surgeon at once.

Because NG tubes often cause sore throat, dry mouth, hoarseness, earache, sore nose, and dry lips, take appropriate nursing measures to combat them. Give your patient frequent gargles of warm tap water or warm saline to relieve his sore throat, and apply lip pomade to both lips and nose to keep the tissues soft. To prevent dehydration from too frequent mouth-rinsing and saliva loss, you might give him some cracked ice to suck. Giving frequent mouth care will prevent parotitis (acute staphylococcus infection of the parotid gland).

A family of Billroths

On the opposite page you'll see three partial gastrectomies. Generally, doctors prefer the Billroth I (Figure 1) because it preserves most of the digestive sequence. The body, antrum, and pylorus of the stomach are removed and the fundus is sutured to the duodenal cuff. Not all patients qualify for a Billroth I, though; one prerequisite is a healthy duodenal cuff that is wide enough for the end-to-end anastomosis. In the Billroth II (Figure 2) the surgeon closes the duodenum and attaches the stump of the stomach to the loop of the jejunum behind the transverse colon (retrocolic). In the antecolic Billroth II procedure (Figure 3) the surgeon closes the duodenum, sutures the remaining stomach to the loop of the jejunum in front of the transverse colon, and anastomoses the afferent and efferent limbs of the jejunum to prevent stasis and rupture in the afferent limb. Whether a surgeon uses the retrocolic or the antecolic procedure, is a matter of his preference.

Other routine postop care includes maintaining hemostasis, observing and recording vital functions, keeping accurate intake and output records, and encouraging ambulation as early as possible — usually on the first postop day.

If your patient undergoes a total gastrectomy, his postoperative care will be similar, but he'll probably recover at a slower rate, depending on how debilitated he was before surgery. He'll have less drainage from his NG tube, because his stomach is no longer present to produce secretions.

If the incision was made in the patient's thoracic cavity, he'll have chest drainage tubes, too. If so, check the amount, color, and consistency of fluid drainage at least once every hour for the first 24 hours after surgery. Check the water-seal chamber for fluctuation and air bubbles; if you note excessive bubbling, notify the doctor at once. Also, check the liquid level in the suction-control chamber to see that it doesn't drop below the level needed to maintain suction. Milk and strip the tube every 1 to 2 hours to keep it patent. And above all, keep the patient comfortable. Chapter 7 explains chest-tube care in detail.

Returning to regular meals — with some restrictions
When the patient's bowel sounds return (usually by the third postop day), indicating that peristalsis has resumed, you can begin giving him clear liquids. Clamp the NG tube and start with 1 ounce of tap water every hour for about 8 hours. Since the patient may be apprehensive, you'll need to give him plenty of encouragement and positive reinforcement. If he tolerates this amount well, increase it to 2 ounces over the next 8 hours, continuing to reinforce and support him psychologically. During this time, observe him closely for signs of abdominal distention, and prepare him for removal of his NG tube. When he's ready physically and psychologically to try oral feedings, the tube can be removed.

After the patient has successfully progressed to liquid feedings, gradually increase his diet to include more fluids and small amounts of soft foods. By about the fifth day after the tube has been removed, he should have progressed to a soft diet of five to six small feedings per day. Never force him to take more than he can tolerate. And always encourage him to chew his foods well to compensate for the loss of his stomach's mixing and liquefying functions.

To prepare the patient for discharge, teach him to select

foods high in protein, low in carbohydrate, moderate in fat, and not too high in bulk. Warn him against eating too much or too fast, as this can cause regurgitation or distention. Generally, the patient will be discharged about the tenth day after surgery.

Overcoming the dumping syndrome and other complications
Numerous complications can follow abdominal surgery — some serious and some not so serious. During the immediate postop period, be particularly alert for signs of these potentially serious complications: hemorrhage from the internal or external suture line, shock, acute tubular necrosis, atelectasis, pneumonia, and fluid or electrolyte imbalance.

During the recovery period, look for secondary hemorrhage from the internal suture line, paralytic ileus (small bowel obstruction), peritonitis and subphrenic abscess, endotoxic shock, pulmonary emboli, cardiac failure, deep-vein thrombosis, wound infection and disruption of abdominal wounds, negative nitrogen balance, external fistula caused by breakdown of the anastomosis, steatorrhea, anemia, and avitaminosis (especially with vitamin B).

A later complication of gastrectomy — after the patient has returned to a regular diet — is the dumping syndrome. This term refers to numerous symptoms that have been classified into two groups: early and late syndrome.

Early dumping syndrome usually occurs with a few minutes after eating and lasts up to 45 minutes. The onset is sudden, and the symptoms include any or all of the following: nausea, weakness, sweating, palpitation, dizziness, flushing, borborygmi, explosive diarrhea, and increased pulse rate and blood pressure. These symptoms may be mild or so severe that they force the patient to lie down.

Late dumping syndrome, which is less serious, occurs 2 to 3 hours after a meal and includes any of the following symptoms: profuse sweating; anxiety; fine tremor of the hands and legs accompanied by vertigo, exhaustion, and lassitude; palpitation; throbbing in the head; faintness; a sensation of hunger; glycosuria; and a marked fall in blood pressure and blood sugar level. Either type of dumping syndrome may last for from 1 year to the rest of the patient's life.

Although many theories have been proposed to explain the dumping syndrome, it still isn't clearly understood. It's proba-

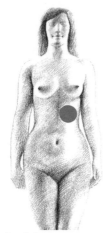

Pathophysiology:
What you should know
Because pancreatic carcinoma is often diagnosed only after it has metastasized, many people underestimate its frequency as a primary site. In truth, pancreatic cancer — when combined with cancer of the biliary tract and the liver — kills twice as many people as stomach cancer. Because its symptoms resemble several benign conditions, pancreatic cancer often isn't discovered until after it has spread to the biliary tract and liver. The two main forms of pancreatic cancer are cylindrical cell (which arises in the ducts and degenerates into cysts) and a large, granular, fatty cell (which arises in the parenchyma). Both form hard, fibrotic nodes; both are highly lethal.

parenchyma). Both form hard, fibrotic nodes; both are highly lethal.

   Cancer of the pancreas metastasizes early and can invade any body organ, but the regional lymph nodes, liver, lungs, and bones are particularly vulnerable.

bly caused by rapid emptying of gastric contents into the small intestine, which has been anastomosed to the gastric stump. Many patients who've had the symptoms have found they can decrease them by avoiding salt, sugar, and high-carbohydrate foods; by taking liquids *between* rather than *with* meals; by eating frequent small meals; and by resting after eating. If the symptoms are severe, surgical intervention may be necessary. This would consist of decreasing the size of the stoma from the stomach into the small intestine to control gastric output.

   Other late complications of gastrectomy are dysphagia, incisional hernia, and symptoms caused by functional, nutritional, and metabolic disorders such as anorexia, hypoproteinemia, and weight loss.

   Complications of the cancer itself include metastasis, recurrence of growth in the stomach, and increased risk that other malignant tumors will develop.

Pancreatic cancer: a bleak outlook
Mr. M.'s recovery from subtotal gastrectomy progressed smoothly, except for a brief episode of dumping syndrome, which was relieved by returning to smaller, more frequent meals. But 6 months later, he went to his family doctor with new complaints. This time he described colicky pain originating in the right hypochondrium and sometimes extending to the subscapular area. He also mentioned vague digestive symptoms (nausea, anexoria), and said he'd lost 10 pounds in 3 weeks.

   A physical examination revealed jaundice, tension, liver enlargement, and palpable gallbladder. Since his pancreas hadn't been removed during the subtotal gastrectomy, his doctor suspected that Mr. M.'s cancer had spread to the pancreas.

   The incidence of pancreatic cancer is increasing and the survival rate, with or without surgery, is bleak. Its cause is unknown, and it's difficult to detect and diagnose. The most common symptom is weight loss. A significant symptom is a dull, aching pain, usually confined to the midepigastrium and frequently radiating to the back. Sitting in a hunched position relieves the pain, but lying on the back accentuates it. Other symptoms include progressive jaundice, pruritis, anorexia, nausea, flatulence, and loss of energy.

   Treatment for cancer of the head of the pancreas is primarily

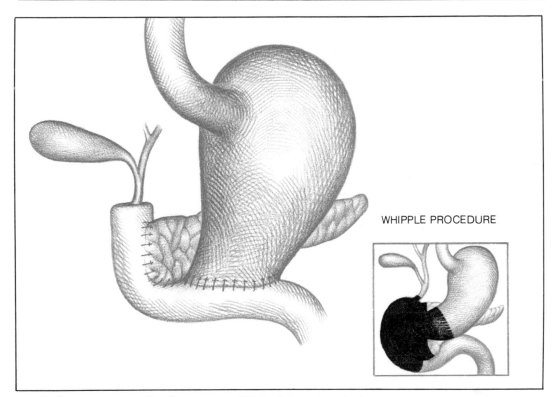

WHIPPLE PROCEDURE

surgical — pancreatoduodenectomy (Whipple's operation). This removes the head and portions of the body and tail of the pancreas, along with the duodenum, a portion of the jejunum, a portion of the stomach, a portion of the pancreatic duct, and the distal portion of the common bile duct. The remaining portions of the stomach, pancreas, and common bile duct are anastomosed to the jejunum (see illustration above).

Patients with pancreatic cancer usually are so debilitated they need 4 to 5 days' preparation for surgery. This includes a high-carbohydrate, high-protein, low-fat diet; oral vitamin supplements; intravenous glucose; and perhaps blood transfusions because of the anemia and depleted blood volume.

The operation is hazardous, with a high mortality rate, and may be done in one or two stages, depending on the patient's physical and emotional status. Postoperatively, the patient is usually acutely ill and his recovery is slow. Postoperative care generally includes maintaining fluid and electrolyte balance, preventing hemorrhage and respiratory complications, maintaining NG tube patency, and providing oral hygiene — plus carefully monitoring vital signs and intake and output.

Pancreatic fistula formation is a frequent and serious complication of pancreatoduodenectomy. Observe the patient's vital signs and wound drainage closely, so you can detect any complications in their early stages.

If most of the pancreas has been removed, the patient will need an oral pancreatic enzyme with meals to aid in digesting fat. He may also need insulin to control endocrine function.

Mr. M. was readmitted to the hospital for a Whipple's operation, which confirmed that his cancer had spread to his pancreas. He tolerated the surgery well and recovered without complications. Upon discharge, he was taking pancreatic enzymes in tablet form, and his jaundice was decreasing. Nevertheless, his prognosis, like that of most patients with pancreatic cancer, is very poor.

Looking ahead
Radiation therapy and chemotherapy haven't been effective in treating stomach or pancreatic cancer to date, although some experiments are being done with 5-FU in treating stomach cancer. Surgery remains the treatment of choice. For you, that means giving these patients good surgical nursing care: relieving pain and discomfort, maintaining adequate nutrition, preventing complications, and preparing them for a smooth convalescence.

With luck, it may cure — and you'll have helped.

SKILLCHECK 3

1. You are a nurse in a physician's office. Mrs. Shapiro's daughter calls, because her mother, a new ostomate, refuses to get dressed and leave the house. Prior to her surgery for cancer of the colon, Mrs. Shapiro was very active in community affairs and an avid golfer. Now the daughter notices that her mother wears too much perfume, and regularly sprays the house with overpowering air fresheners. What can you do?

2. Sheila Katz, a 42-year-old mother of two, had a 1 cm noninvasive tumor in the rectosigmoid, which the surgeon treated with a wide resection and anastamosis.

   Mrs. Katz has incisional pain, which inhibits her breathing and leg exercises, and getting her to ambulate after the surgery requires much coaxing. Three days postop, she refuses to get out of bed because of leg pains. She has a fever. What do you do?

3. Red Taggart is a 50-year-old insurance agent, who is making a slow recovery from a total gastrectomy for advanced stomach cancer. His nasogastric tube is still in place 3 days postop, though drainage is slight and he has no abdominal distention. This morning, Mr. Taggart complains of a sore throat, but you know his physician doesn't plan to remove the tube and start him on oral feedings for several days. What can you do to make him more comfortable?

4. Tom Graves is a 60-year-old factory worker, who has worked the night shift for the past 25 years. He is 10 days postop a resection for cancer of the sigmoid colon. He and his wife are still somewhat confused about the surgery, but he is slowly learning to care for his colostomy. Soon he will be returning to work. How can you tailor his colostomy care to fit his schedule?

5. You have just administered pain medication to Ralph Mott, a 56-year-old plumber, who is 2 days postop a Billroth II gastrectomy for stomach cancer. Twenty minutes later, his wife appears at the desk with the complaint that he seems "uncomfortable," even though he is asleep. What should you do?

6. On the 4th of July, 60-year-old Albert Johnson, who is 6 weeks postop a gastrectomy for stomach cancer, is rushed to the emergency room with severe abdominal cramps. He is weak, perspiring freely, and complains of dizziness. A check of his vital signs reveals a high pulse rate and elevated blood pressure. You ask his anxious wife for more details and she begins by telling you that they spent the afternoon with their grandchildren. What do you ask next?

7. Maria Buckwalter is a 54-year-old English teacher, who is 3 days postop an abdominal perineal resection for cancer of the rectum. Sometime during the night, her colostomy appliance became too full and pulled away from her stoma bud, causing serosanguineous drainage to leak on her abdomen. The skin around Ms. Buckwalter's stoma is excoriated and she is very upset. What do you do?

(Answers on page 179)

CARING FOR PATIENTS WITH CANCER OF THE PELVIS

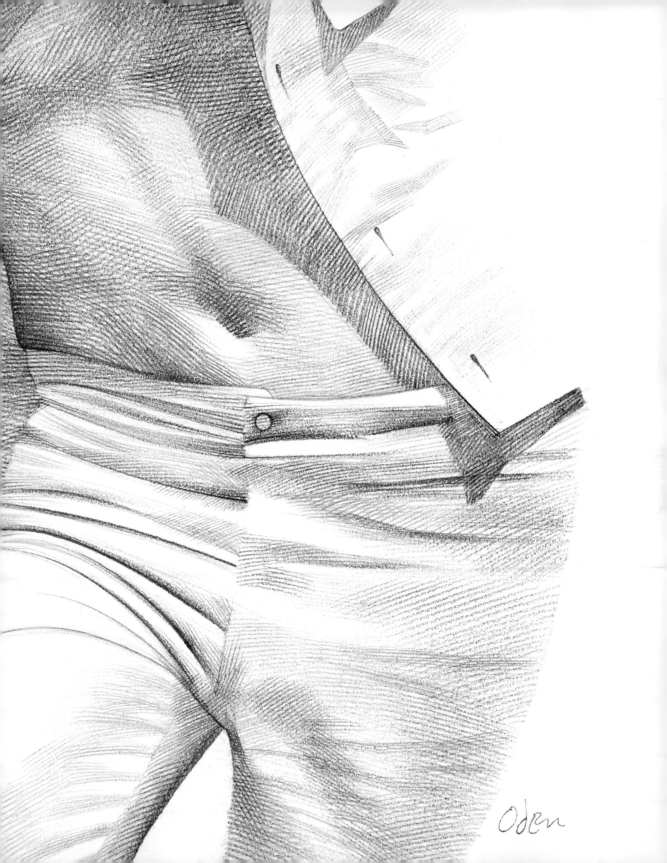

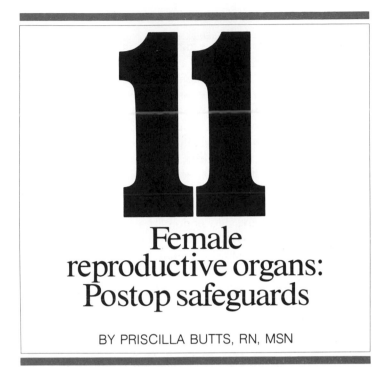

11

Female reproductive organs: Postop safeguards

BY PRISCILLA BUTTS, RN, MSN

NURSING CARE OF WOMEN with cancer of the reproductive organs creates a special problem. No matter what surgery she has — or how far the cancer is advanced — you may identify with her, if you're a woman. If she chooses a pelvic exenteration to palliate the ravages of the disease, you may be affected emotionally, and that may hamper the quality of your nursing care. Can you keep the quality high, still maintaining a positive attitude? What about the complications that may occur after a pelvic exenteration or hysterectomy? Can you recognize and treat hemorrhage from a perineal wound, infection in the abdominal incision or ileal conduit, or rectovaginal fistula? This chapter tells you how to do these things and more. It'll tell you what to expect — from the time of the patient's diagnosis to discharge — and help you and the patient cope.

Definitive diagnosing

The cancer's original location and extent of its invasion determine the treatment: surgery, radiation, chemotherapy, or a combination. But a complete diagnostic workup is needed to give the physician this information. He may already suspect cancer, of course, from the results of a patient's Pap smear or

Pathophysiology:
What you should know

Cancer of female reproductive organs may be 1 of 4 major types. UTERINE CERVIX. Ninety-five per cent of these lesions arise from the epithelium of the cervical lips or canal as epidermoid or squamous cell carcinomas. Exophytic tumors infiltrate the vaginal canal; endophytic infiltrate the entire cervix; and ulcerating involve the vaginal fornices. In any case, the first signs may be vaginal discharge and bleeding. Cervical cancer spreads slowly, to the vaginal fornices and wall, uterine body, parametria, regional lymph nodes, and bladder and rectum. ENDOMETRIUM. Tumors of this site are usually well differentiated adenocarcinomas that arise anywhere in the endometrial epithelium. The disease spreads slowly to the regional lymph nodes and the lower part of the vagina. First signs mimic those of cervical cancer.
OVARIES. Forty per cent of these tumors are cystadenomas which, though benign, can become malignant. Other tumors include mesenchymal with hormone activity, germinomas, teratomas, and tumors of the ovarian stroma. Usually these produce no early signs or symptoms. Ovarian tumors spread to the regional lymph nodes and, in advanced stages, to the lungs and liver. VULVA. Eighty per cent of these primary lesions are well differentiated epidermoid epitheliomas, mostly ulcerogranulating. The lesions most frequently occur in the labia majora, then the labia minora, the clitoris, and the posterior commissure. The earliest sign is pruritis. Vulvar cancer spreads to the vagina and the regional lymph nodes. In advanced stages it may overtake the lungs, liver, and bones.

pelvic examination. To get a more definitive diagnosis, the patient will be hospitalized for a biopsy. The physician may also do a metastatic X-ray evaluation and a sigmoidoscopy to see if the cancer involves the colon.

Consider the case of Mrs. W., a 43-year-old mother of four, who went to her doctor for abnormal vaginal bleeding. When her Pap smear showed cervical cancer, she was admitted to the hospital for a more definitive diagnosis. If her cancer had been confined to the cervix, she may have had a radium implant to keep the cancer from spreading to the vagina, then a complete hysterectomy. However, a jet wash done soon after she was admitted revealed endometrial cancer. Mrs. W.'s treatment plan was revised, and she was given external radiation (instead of an implant) to keep the cancer from infiltrating her lymphatic system.

Sometimes a physician specifies internal radiation, despite evidence of the cancer's spread. This may happen when the patient is too debilitated from the advanced cancer to tolerate external radiation. But, radiation of any kind can cause serious problems for the patient with cancer of the female reproductive organs: For example, she may develop an ulceration around the implant, a recto- or vesicovaginal fistula, or an intestinal obstruction. Later in this chapter, we'll see how to recognize fistulae. For a complete discussion of radiation and its side effects, see Chapter 4.

Why a pelvic exenteration?

Mrs. W. was relatively lucky, because her cancer had not invaded other organs in the pelvic cavity. Some patients are not this lucky, and may be admitted to the hospital for recurrent pelvic cancer some time after initial treatment with a hysterectomy. When the cancer is this far advanced, the patient may undergo screening tests to see if she's a candidate for a full or partial pelvic exenteration. If tests show her cancer has metastasized to other parts of the body (e.g., breast, brain, bone), and she's severely cachetic, the surgeon may decide against such extensive surgery. An exenteration doesn't necessarily extend the life of every patient with pelvic cancer, even when there's no evidence of distant metastases.

Such surgery is palliative, though, and reduces much of the pain the patient would feel in the terminal stages of her disease. That's why many patients are willing to undergo this radical

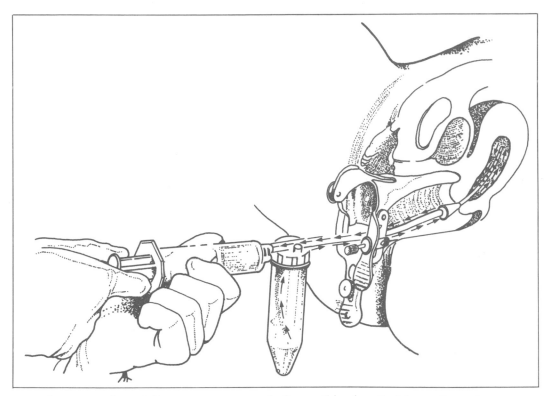

procedure, even though it may mean removal of everything in their pelvic cavity, including the vagina, and construction of an ileal conduit and colostomy. You must accept the disappointment a patient feels if she's turned down, no matter what your attitude is about this mutilating surgery. The patient has a right to cling to life as long as possible, and may feel it's being taken away from her if she's rejected for a pelvic exenteration.

Which surgery for Mrs. W.?

Mrs. W.'s cancer, however, appeared to be confined to her reproductive organs. So, her treatment would be preop radiation, then a hysterectomy and bilateral salpingo-oophorectomy. We prepared her for the surgery by explaining everything that would happen to her in the O.R. and afterwards. We encouraged her to talk about her cancer and verbalize her fears about dying (see Chapter 3 for tips). We discussed what she'd heard about hysterectomies, to sort out any misinformation.

Deriving a diagnosis

Doctors may use the following methods to reach a diagnosis:
BIOPSY (ENDOMETRIAL). The walls of the endometrium are scraped (curretage) and studied under a microscope.
BIOPSY (CERVICAL). The cervix is painted with an iodine solution, which leaves only the abnormal cells unstained. Abnormal cells are biopsied and examined by a pathologist.
COLPOSCOPY. With this diagnostic procedure, changes in the vascular pattern of the cervix and vaginal vault can be seen.
JET WASH (see figure above). Isotonic saline is forced into the uterus through a cannula and withdrawn, carrying cells from the endometrium. These are examined under a microscope.

A lexicon of exenterations
Figure 1 on the opposite page shows the normal pelvic organs. Pelvic exenteration may be partial, retaining an unaffected colorectum (Figure 2) or an unaffected bladder (Figure 3), or if all the organs are cancerous, it may be total (Figure 4).

Patients don't always understand their anatomy as well as they should. For example, a patient may realize she'll have her ovaries removed during an oophorectomy, but doesn't understand that she'll go into her menopause (if she hasn't already). You must be careful to remind her of this, but at the same time reassure her that she won't look different after the surgery or lose her interest in sex. Mrs. W.'s main concern, quite naturally, was the cancer. We spoke positively about her chance for a cure and reassured her family.

What kind of physical preparation did Mrs. W. need preoperatively? First, she had routine laboratory tests, including a check for nutritional deficiencies. When a patient has a protein deficiency, as many cancer patients do, she'll be started on a high-protein diet, and — in some cases — surgery will be delayed. (For more details on patients with protein deficiencies, see Chapter 3.)

The night before surgery, we prepped Mrs. W. by giving her a cleansing enema, and by shaving and scrubbing her abdomen with antibacterial soap. We applied antiembolism stockings to prevent thrombophlebitis. These would remain in place while she was in the hospital, although they would be changed periodically to maintain proper circulation.

After surgery, Mrs. W. needed all the attention usually given to a patient after abdominal surgery. She returned from the recovery room with an I.V. and Foley catheter. Unlike the I.V., which is normally removed when the patient has stabilized, the catheter stays in place for about 2 days. Mrs. W. was then given a chance to void naturally. If she hadn't been able to, we would have recatheterized her. Voiding can be a big problem for the patient whose bladder has been traumatized by surgery.

Mrs. W. complained of gas pains 2 days postop — a common difficulty for patients after abdominal surgery. We gave her an antiflatulent (Mylicon, Phazyme) and encouraged her to walk around more often. We watched for evidence of nausea or vomiting along with abdominal distention, signs of a paralytic ileus. If they'd occurred, we'd have put her back on clear liquids and called the physician. If she'd developed chest pains, we'd have checked for a pulmonary embolus or myocardial infarction. Then we'd have administered oxygen, if needed, ordered a stat EKG, and called the physician.

With patients like this, you must be alert for an incisional

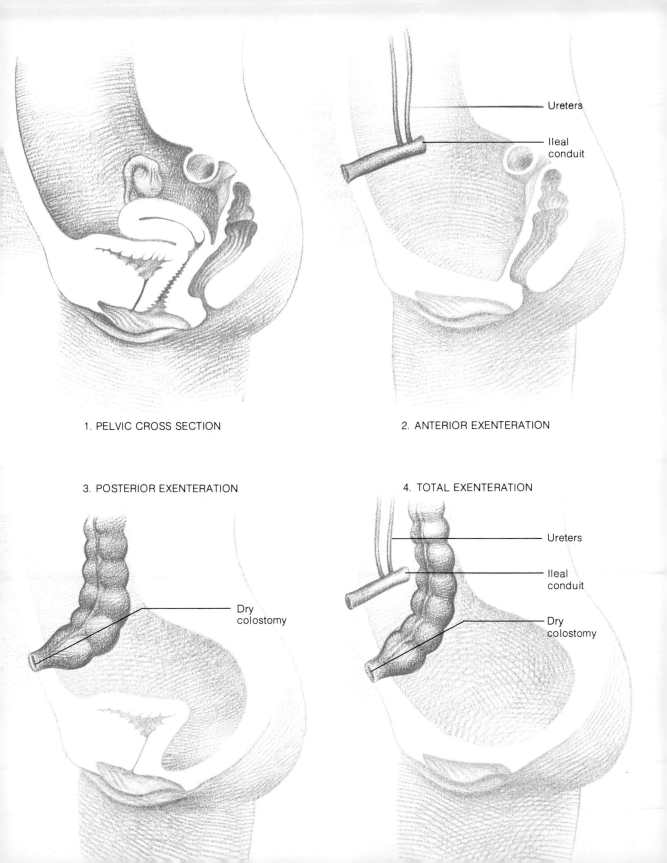

1. PELVIC CROSS SECTION

2. ANTERIOR EXENTERATION

Ureters

Ileal conduit

3. POSTERIOR EXENTERATION

Dry colostomy

4. TOTAL EXENTERATION

Ureters

Ileal conduit

Dry colostomy

infection. It's one of the most serious postop problems after a hysterectomy or pelvic exenteration.

We suspected an incisional infection when Mrs. W. complained of distention and discomfort in that area. And we noticed slight dehiscence and foul-smelling, purulent drainage. So, we cultured the drainage promptly and notified the physician, who soon started Mrs. W. on antibiotics. Then we cleaned around the infected area with povidone-iodine (Betadine) and applied warm compresses (using sterile water) for 20 minutes, four times a day. Each time we removed the compresses, we put a clean dressing over the incision.

Still another serious problem a cancer patient may have after a hysterectomy is a recto- or vesicovaginal fistula. These can be caused by radiation damage to the tissues from an implant. You suspect a rectovaginal fistula when feces drain into the vagina; a vesicovaginal fistula when the drainage is urine. Treating a fistula in a patient whose tissue is already deteriorated by cancer is very difficult. A pelvic exenteration would eliminate the possibility of having painful fistulae in the terminal stages of the disease. That's one reason why a patient would choose exenteration.

Mrs. W. was discharged from our hospital 8 days postop. But, before she left we reminded her that she'd be going into her menopause, and might experience the symptoms: hot flashes, night sweats and vaginal dryness. We urged her to notify her physician if these symptoms occurred so he could start her on hormonal replacement therapy if he hasn't already. We also taught her breast self-examination (see Chapter 8) and stressed the need for regular checkups. The patient who's had a hysterectomy for cancer of the uterus should have a Pap smear of the vagina every 6 months; cancer cells may have shed into the vaginal area.

When the patient has a pelvic exenteration

What about the patient who has a pelvic exenteration? She may already have had a total hysterectomy. So she won't need psychological preparation for her menopause, as Mrs. W. did. But she and her family will need a great deal of emotional support to face the treatment chosen.

What are your own feelings about this extensive surgery? Many nurses have difficulty accepting it as an alternative. See things from the patient's point of view, if you can, and try to

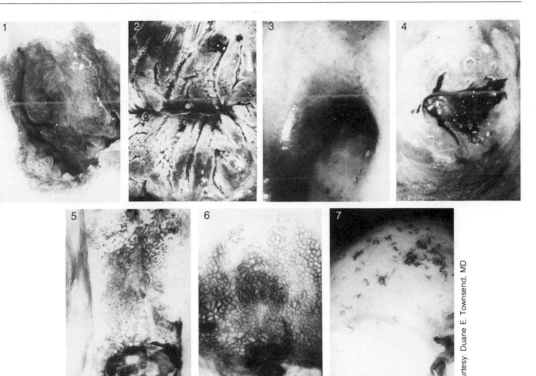

Courtesy: Duane E. Townsend, MD

Conditions of the cervix

In many women, a portion of the exocervix and the endocervical canal is covered with columnar epithelium having a grape-like appearance, while the remainder of the cervix is covered by smooth squamous epithelium. The interface between these two types of tissue is called the *squamo-columnar junction* (see Fig. 1). About 90 to 95% of squamous cancers of the cervix begin at the squamocolumnar junction.

With the beginning of menstruation, changes in a woman's hormone balance and in the vaginal pH stimulate a process whereby columnar epithelium is gradually replaced by squamous epithelium. This process, called *squamous metaplasia* (see Fig. 2), occurs

both as a peripheral ingrowth from the squamocolumnar junction and as islands of metaplasia within the transformation zone. In most women, metaplasia progresses as a normal process. Mature, normal, smooth squamous epithelium gradually covers the entire exocervix and extends into the endocervical canal, forming a *normal trans-formation zone* (see Fig. 3). The colposcopic examination focuses on this transformation zone.

But in a few women, a change toward anaplasia begins and abnormal squamous epithelium develops within the transformation zone. An atypical transformation zone has one or more of the following abnormal colposcopic findings:

- *White epithelium* — a

transient phenomenon that shows up after the acetic acid test in areas of increased nuclear density (see Fig. 4).
- *Punctation* — a stippled pattern of the cervical capillaries (see Fig. 5).
- *Mosaic* — a mosaic pattern of the vascular network of the cervix (see Fig. 6).
- *Abnormal vessels* — irregular vessels with abrupt courses resembling commas, corkscrews, or spaghetti-like forms (see Fig. 7).

Abnormal findings by themselves don't indicate a diagnosis of cancer or even precancerous lesions. They do indicate the need to have that area biopsied. A colposcopically directed biopsy can provide a more definitive diagnosis.

Pain: A progressive path
Cervical cancer has slipped into second place among pain-producing cancers. Still, the pain of cervical cancer in the terminal stages commands attention. Usually it is progressive, starting in the lumbar region, extending to the hip and thigh, and stopping temporarily at the knee. In the late stages, it extends all the way to the ankle and toes. Although the severity varies from patient to patient, a general rule holds that the more extensive the tumor is, the more intense and extensive the pain. If the tumor invades the anterior vaginal wall or the bladder, it can cause suprapubic pain. Contrary to popular belief, the pain of cervical cancer only rarely is related to rectovaginal fistulae.

understand why she has chosen it. Be positive and reassuring as you explain everything that will happen to her postoperatively. Teach her about the ileal conduit and/or colostomy she will have (see Chapters 9 and 13 for details), and make sure she understands that the surgeon will remove her vagina. (If she's sexually active, he may make an attempt later to reconstruct the vagina with plastic surgery.)

The bowel and skin preparation before pelvic exenteration is much more extensive than for hysterectomy. The danger of infection is greater, because the surgery involves the colon, where there are large amounts of bacteria.

First, the patient goes on a low-residue diet 48 to 72 hours before surgery, then a clear liquid diet the last day before she's permitted nothing by mouth. The physician will order an oral antibiotic like kanamycin sulfate, a cathartic, and one or more cleansing enemas, possibly an antibiotic added to them. The night before surgery, you'll prep the patient's abdomen and perineal area with antibacterial soap. You may have been doing this daily from the time of the patient's admittance, because some surgeons order it.

An enterostomal specialist may see the patient before surgery to mark the skin for stoma placement.

Pelvic exenteration is, of course, much more extensive than a hysterectomy. The patient will return from the O.R. with many tubes and drains to maintain: a nasogastric tube, I.V. and CVP line, a Hemovac in the incision to drain and prevent peritoneal distention, and temporary stoma bags to catch initial fecal and urine drainage. Her unsutured perineal wound will be packed with sterile gauze, and her abdominal incision dressings will be held in place with a T or Montgomery strap binder. Depending on her condition, the patient may also be on a respirator. Monitor her closely and control her pain. In our hospital, the medications frequently prescribed for pain control are hydroxyzine hydrochloride (Vistaril), and hydromorphone (Dilaudid). We also place the patient on Puff Packs, inserted between the sheet and mattress. (An air mattress can also help relieve discomfort.) We give her all the emotional support we can at this difficult time, and reassure her family.

When you're caring for stomas, incision, and perineal wound, watch the amount and color of the patient's drainage carefully. A change can be the first sign of a dangerous infection or life-threatening hemorrhage. Be especially alert for signs of hemorrhage when the surgeon removes the perineal wound packing about 48 to 72 hours postoperatively. Some bright red bleeding always appears at first, but this should never be excessive. Check the pads you've placed under the patient's perineal area. If she's soaking them through, call the physician immediately.

You can expect normal drainage from the perineal wound to be heavy and serosanguineous the first few days. But gradually, the color will lighten to a straw color, and the amount will decrease as the wound closes. If it changes back to bright red, notify the physician immediately.

Bleeding from the ileal conduit can mean an anastamosis didn't heal properly; the patient will have to return to the O.R. for surgical revision. Also be alert for bleeding from the stoma sites and from the abdominal incision of a patient with a pelvic exenteration or hysterectomy. Bleeding from an incision could indicate that the internal suture line has ruptured, and the patient may have dehiscence followed by evisceration.

Foul-smelling, purulent drainage from a stoma or perineal wound can signify a serious infection. If you discover that, culture the drainage and notify the physician. He will start the patient on antibiotics piggybacked with an I.V. of 150 cc D_5W. Caution: A patient with an incisional or anastamosis infection may develop peritonitis. Be alert for these symptoms: elevated temperature; pain; rigid, distended abdomen; labored breathing; increased pulse rate; and diminished or absent bowel sounds. Call the physician at once.

Proper care of skin and perineal wound postoperatively obviously helps to prevent infection. Be sure to keep the skin clean after pelvic exenteration, because there'll be so much fecal and urine drainage. Clean the perineal wound several times a day with a warm saline-and-water solution. You can teach the patient to use a Sitz bath for this when she is ambulatory. You may need to assist her, however, to make sure she irrigates the entire perineal area. (Obese patients may have difficulty doing this without help.) Use a heat lamp to dry the wound area.

Going home with hope
Teaching your patient self-care before she's discharged from the hospital will speed her recovery from this extensive surgery. This teaching should include showing how to care for

her own stomas and explaining the possibility of vaginal re-construction. If you're comfortable discussing the subject, you may suggest other means of sexual gratification to her — but make sure *she* feels comfortable discussing the subject before you bring it up.

Caring for a woman with cancer of the reproductive organs can be extremely difficult, especially when it's so far advanced that she's chosen a pelvic exenteration. Besides all the physical problems you'll encounter, your feelings as a person are involved. You may identify with her. Don't let this affect the quality of your nursing care. Be as positive as you can with your patient; together, you draw from each other's strengths.

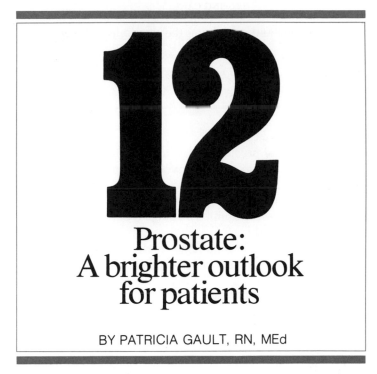

12

Prostate:
A brighter outlook
for patients

BY PATRICIA GAULT, RN, MEd

CANCER OF THE PROSTATE. For the patient, this diagnosis can mean surgery, impotence, possible incontinence, and maybe death. For you as his nurse, it means caring for the many problems that can accompany the disease: excessive bleeding, possible hemorrhage, bladder spasms, and infection.

Combatting a killer
Prostate cancer is the most common cancer in men over 50, and it occurs in about 50% of men over 75. It rates third as a killer from cancer in men. Even so, the outlook is getting brighter for its victims, thanks to early detection, radical surgery, hormone therapy, and antineoplastics. Your patient's treatment will depend on his age, health, and the extent of his cancer.

Many patients with prostate cancer come to the hospital because of urinary obstruction, which is removed with a resectoscope during a transurethral resection (TUR). The tissue is then examined by a pathologist to confirm the diagnosis of cancer. If the patient is over 65 with prostate cancer, sometimes little is done after the TUR — he's just made more comfortable with an orchiectomy and hormonal therapy.

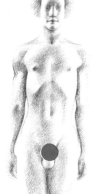

**Pathophysiology:
What you should know**
Prostate cancers are adenocarcinomas that vary in appearance and differentiation. They arise most commonly in the posterior lobe, occasionally in the anterior lobe, and almost never in the median lobe. An early sign of prostate cancer is dysuria; later signs include chronic urinary retention with dribbling, edema of the legs and, in late metastasis, palpable edema of the skull, ribs, and clavicles. Prostate cancer spreads locally by infiltration to the bladder, seminal vesicles, and peritoneum. Distant metastases by the bloodstream and lymph system affect the bones, especially the vertebrae, pelvis, femora, and ribs.

More radical surgery is usually ordered for victims under age 65 with no evidence of metastasis. A surgeon may remove a cancerous prostate with a retropubic or perineal prostatectomy (see Figures on page 134). Of these, the perineal is the most common.

The radical approaches

A radical perineal prostatectomy was done with Mr. S., age 55, whose cancer appeared to involve the prostate, and also both posterior lobes with extension to the seminal vesicles. Scans of liver, lung, and bone showed no evidence of metastasis; his cancer was classified as Stage C or III, depending on the staging system.

How do you care for a patient life Mr. S.? Before surgery, you usually administer an enema with an antibiotic to prevent fecal contamination of the operative site. You also put antiembolism stockings on his legs.

Postoperatively, stay alert for many problems. If trouble is going to arise after prostatic surgery, it usually will do so in the first 24 hours. Check your patient's vital signs every 2 hours, paying particular attention to a pulse rate falling below 60 beats per minutes — bradycardia. This may be due to prolonged spinal anesthesia and calls for atropine, I.V. or I.M., to stimulate the sluggish beat.

Record your patient's oral temperature every 4 hours the first day. If it's over 101° F. (38.3° C.), that may mean infection. Watch for signs of hemorrhage, which can easily occur because of the lesion's increased vascularity. With Mr. S., we noticed copious amounts of urine draining from the perineal drain; drainage from the Foley catheter diminished as the perineal flow increased. You have to anticipate skin problems when this occurs and use a T-binder (instead of tape) to hold the dressings in place. Cover dressings with a disposable diaper before you fasten the T-binder.

Change the dressings and diaper hourly and weigh them to figure the exact amount of drainage from the perineal wound. To do this, subtract the dry weight and calculate that 1 gram of weight equals 1 cc of fluid.

Sometimes, for a large amount of drainage, the urologist will apply traction to the catheter and order an antispasmodic against any subsequent bladder spasms. As drainage diminishes, you'll notice a gradual increase of urine from the catheter. When drainage ceases, the doctor removes the drain.

Because Mr. S. received propantheline bromide (Pro-Banthine) for bladder spasms, he developed a paralytic ileus. So, we maintained the I.V. fluids and kept him NPO for several more days.

Never give enemas or suppositories to your patient after radical perineal surgery; you may contaminate the wound. When he can take fluids, start him on a low-residue diet and give oral laxatives. Cleanse his wound with povidone-iodine (Betadine) after each BM to prevent infection.

Fecal contamination of the wound site generally isn't a problem after a suprapubic or retropubic prostatectomy, but many of these other complications occur, so watch your patient closely.

A radical prostatectomy of any type leaves most patients impotent and some of them permanently incontinent. You'll need to help them and their families cope with this distressing news after the urologist discusses it with them. Some patients adjust fairly well; others need a lot of emotional support.

Sometimes, the physician can help the patient achieve continence after surgery by prescribing perineal exercises and bethanechol chloride (Urecholine) to improve bladder tone. If micturition control seems unlikely during his hospital stay, keep the patient as dry as possible so he can socialize with his family and friends without embarrassment.

TUR troubles

Occasionally, you'll have a patient like Mr. D., whose cystoscopy revealed a nonresectable cancerous lesion of the prostate. His obstruction was removed transurethrally with a resectoscope, and he returned from the O.R. with a Foley catheter inserted in his bladder and continuous irrigation. (Usually, a continuous drip of irrigation is enough to cleanse the bladder and reduce the chance of clot formation.) With a patient like Mr. D., you check his irrigation returns every hour or more often the first day. Look for changes in vital signs, increasing pallor, or bloody drainage.

How do you control excessive bleeding which can occur almost any time after surgery? You can tell excessive bleeding because urine returns darken suddenly. Ordinarily, fluid draining into the collection bag lightens from reddish pink to light pink within 24 hours, or more.

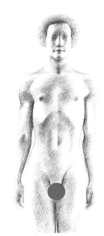

Pathophysiology:
What you should know
Most testicular cancers arise from germ tissue: About 80% are seminogoniomas and spermatocyte seminomas, while about 20% are dysembryomas. Those containing trophoblasts secrete gonadotrophins and may involve gynecomastia and feminization. Firmness and differentiation of the tumors vary, as does size — some enlarge the organ up to 10 times its original size, while others remain small. Hemorrhage and necrosis often develop, but usually the first sign of a testicular tumor is abdominal distress.

Because of the complicated lymphatic network surrounding the testes, testicular cancers may metastasize while the primary tumor remains small. The disease spreads to the regional lymph nodes, the lungs, and the liver but rarely to the bone.

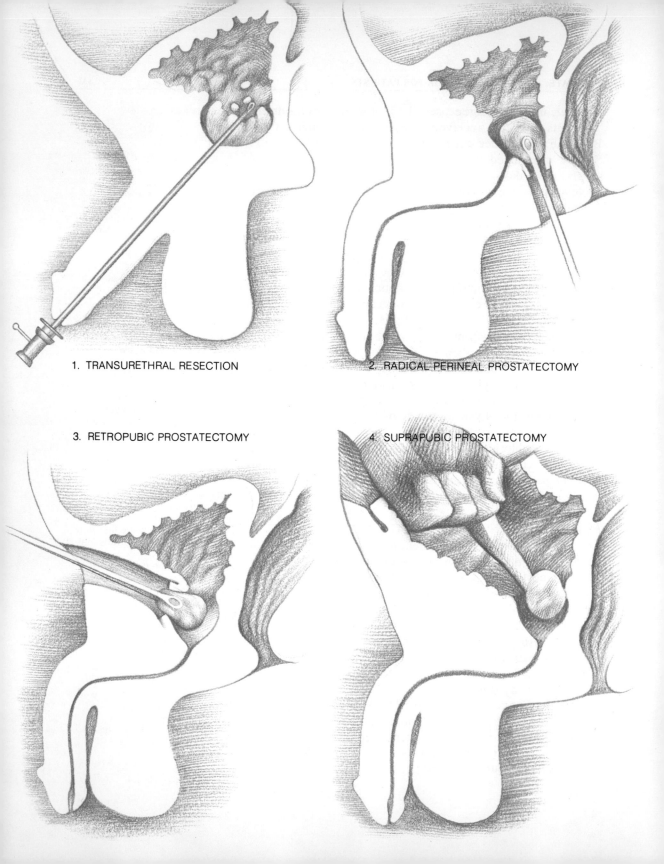

1. TRANSURETHRAL RESECTION

2. RADICAL PERINEAL PROSTATECTOMY

3. RETROPUBIC PROSTATECTOMY

4. SUPRAPUBIC PROSTATECTOMY

You can often tell the type of bleeding from the return's color. If it's bright red with increased viscosity and numerous clots, that usually means arterial blood, especially if the patient's blood pressure falls. If it's darker and less viscous, that usually means venous bleeding (more common). You can usually control venous bleeding on the spot; arterial hemorrhage will send the patient back to the O.R. for further cautery.

To identify Mr. D.'s type of bleeding we increased the irrigation, but the flow didn't dislodge any clots or alter color. A few small clots appeared moments later, when we irrigated his catheter with normal saline using a Toomey syringe.

We reconnected the continuous drip. When the returns stayed dark (indicating venous bleeding), the urologist asked me to try to stop the bleeding by applying traction. (Not all urologists will permit nurses to apply traction, but many will let more experienced nurses do it. With traction, the ballooned end of the catheter inside the bladder applies pressure to the prostatic fossa.) Several hours later, after Mr. D.'s drainage lightened, I released traction, and no further bleeding occurred. You rarely maintain traction longer than 24 hours because of potential trauma to the external urinary sphincter.

Watch for signs of bladder spasms, which can result from irritation by the catheter balloon, especially in patients requiring traction. Spasms can also result from bladder distention, a frequent occurrence when a catheter clogs. If your patient complains of pain and the need to "move his bowels and urinate at the same time," suspect bladder spasms. Look for the cause by shutting off the irrigation and palpating his lower abdomen for a distended bladder. Is the catheter clogged? Try to clear it. If gentle suction dislodges any accumulated clots or tissue remnants, irrigate the catheter again after the saline initially instilled has drained out. Repeat at least every 4 hours until the drainage is free of clots. If the catheter doesn't clear, the urologist will remove it and insert another.

Some patients are given belladonna and opium suppositories to decrease pain from bladder spasms. Propantheline bromide is equally effective. Many urologists order antispasmodics prophylactically for patients requiring traction, because it can trigger spasms. But, caution: Patients with severe cardiac disease or glaucoma shouldn't get these drugs, — they increase heart rate and intraocular pressure. Also, antispasmodic drugs can cause constipation, so prevent this

Prostate procedures

A transurethral resection (TUR) of the prostate (see Figure 1 on the opposite page) is performed to relieve the patient's presenting symptom of urethral obstruction. Alert to the possibility of cancer, the surgeon first examines the gland with a cystoscope, then uses a resectoscope to remove the obstruction. (If prostate cancer is suspected without obstruction, the surgeon may perform a transperineal or transrectal biopsy with a Silvermann needle.) If the tissue sample reveals cancer, the surgeon may recommend additional radical surgery to excise the remaining gland.

In one of these surgical procedures, the radical perineal prostatectomy (Figure 2), the surgeon incises the posterior prostatic fossa through an incision anterior to the rectum and removes the prostatic capsule, the seminal vesicles, and the bladder neck.

In a mirror image of the perineal approach, the retropubic prostatectomy (Figure 3) is performed through an incision in the lower abdomen. The surgeon opens the anterior prostatic capsule and enucleates the enlarged gland. If he discovers that it's malignant, he'll remove the capsule, seminal vesicles, and bladder neck through the same incision.

In a suprapubic prostatectomy (Figure 4) the surgeon opens the bladder and enucleates the prostate with his finger. This procedure is performed mostly for benign lesions, but if the surgeon finds cancer, he'll recommend more radical surgery.

Pain: Later than you'd think
Despite their appearance, testicular tumors usually cause little more than discomfort in the early stages. Later, they might cause a dull ache. And in the advanced stage they may cause lumbar pain, which radiates down to the thigh and throughout the sciatic nerve distribution.

complication by giving the patient a stool softener.

Mr. D.'s cancer, as we said earlier, was nonresectable. So his TUR was followed by a bilateral scrotal orchiectomy (removal of the testicles through an incision in the scrotal sac).

When your patient has an orchiectomy, watch for bleeding and swelling. Relieve his minor discomfort with a mild analgesic. Applying ice packs to the scrotal area the first day may also help. If the patient is ambulatory, suggest an athletic supporter. Usually, absorbable sutures close the incision, so expect only minimal drainage when you remove the gauze dressings the day after surgery. Report profuse drainage.

Sometimes a wound infection occurs after an orchiectomy. This happened with Mr. D., whose temperature rose to 102° F. (38.9° C.). His scrotum was swollen and tender. We notified the urologist promptly and he opened the suture line, inserting a drain. We applied hot packs to the area and administered ampicillin trihydrate orally. This was continued for 10 days, until the infection subsided.

After an orchiectomy, a patient with nonresectable prostate cancer may have cobalt treatments and oral diethylstilbestrol. Diethylstilbestrol usually causes the patient to gain weight, get a softer beard, and develop enlarged breasts. To reduce the chance of enlargement, radiotherapy to the breast area may be given before diethylstilbestrol treatment.

Your patient may experience other side effects from daily doses of diethylstilbestrol. Nausea is one, so try to give it just before bedtime. Never give diethylstilbestrol or diethylstilbestrol diphosphate to patients with signs of congestive heart failure: peripheral edema, shortness of breath, productive cough, and weight gain. Notify the doctor if you see these signs. He may decide to give the drug anyway, to decrease pain in patients with metastasized cancer.

Chemotherapy has prolonged the lives of many prostate cancer patients (see Chapter 5), and improved antineoplastics are being developed every year with promising results. One of these is cis-Platinum, currently undergoing trials.

The next patient you care for may have prostate cancer. He may have problems with excessive bleeding, hemorrhage, bladder spasms, and infection. What you've learned from this chapter will help you cope with these difficulties. You can give him the physical care he needs — and by truly empathizing, the emotional support he and his family need.

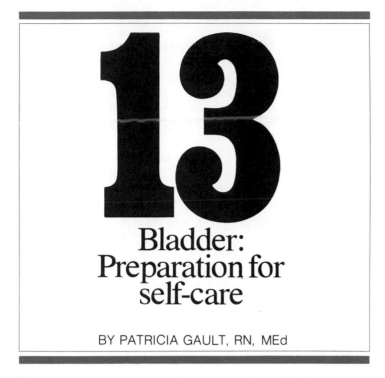

13

Bladder: Preparation for self-care

BY PATRICIA GAULT, RN, MEd

CARING FOR A PATIENT with cancer of the bladder means dealing with his physical needs, true, but it also means dealing with his emotional ones. For, like the patient with colorectal cancer, he may face drastic alteration of body image through construction of a stoma on the abdominal wall. And, for a man, surgery means facing impotence coming from the removal of the seminal vesicles and the prostate.

Only by getting to know the patient's personal characteristics can you give him the best care. And only by teaching him (and his family) to care for the stoma and to deal with his altered body image, can you help him come back to a productive life.

One of the group
Actually patients with carcinoma of the bladder fall into two distinct groups. The first, those with noninvasive bladder cancer, simply have the tumor resected through a cystoscope and then return periodically for examination. Any recurrent tumor is resected each time.

The other group, those whose cancer invades the muscle wall or beyond, may be scheduled for more radical surgery —

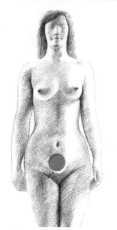

Pathophysiology: What you should know

The most common tumor of the urinary bladder, transitional cell carcinoma, arises from the transitional epithelium of the mucous membrane. The tumors may be solid, ulcerative, or fronded; single or multiple; infiltrating or non-infiltrating. Whatever the structure, they probably will cause painless hematuria.

Bladder tumors may remain localized for a long time, but the most pernicious soon spread to the regional lymph nodes, bones, lungs, and liver. Some tumors spread directly into the pelvic tissues.

removal of the bladder and construction of a stoma — or a combined form of treatment (including surgery, radiation, and chemotherapy). These patients may come from the first group after passage of time or they may be patients who notice some telltale sign — usually blood in the urine — that sends them to the urologist for perhaps their first visit. A typical patient was Mrs. W., 61.

When Mrs. W. noted blood in her urine, she saw her personal physician, who prescribed sulfizoxazole (Gantrisin). After the hematuria returned a few weeks later, she was admitted for further evaluation. Mrs. W. had no dysuria or other changes in her urinary pattern, and the urine culture and some other tests turned out to be negative. But painless, gross hematuria in a 61-year-old woman (her urinalysis revealed 50-100 RBC/HPF [high power field] and a large amount of hemoglobin) suggested bladder carcinoma. (Bloody urine is the first sign in about 60% of all bladder tumors.) And the intravenous pyelogram showed a questionable shadow in the bladder.

During cystoscopy, the urologist found a 3-centimeter tumor on the anterior bladder wall. This was resected and removed through the urethra and the specimen was sent to the pathologist. The pathologist's report revealed a Grade III tumor, one that had already invaded the muscle wall. Luckily, liver and bone scans and full lung tomograms showed no evidence of metastasis.

The urologist talked over the biopsy results and their meaning with Mrs. W., gave her a week to settle some family matters, and sent her to the radiologist for four cobalt treatments delivering a total of 1600 rads to the pelvis. A combination of radiotherapy and surgery are now often used, for recent research has shown that preoperative radiation improves the overall chances of survival. (When the cancer is so extensive that no other treatment is possible, external radiation may be used as the sole treatment. Radiation in such a case is only palliative, however.)

Clearing the system

The patient who is to have a bladder resection is given antibiotics by mouth along with enemas to reduce the chance of infection from bowel flora. After she was admitted on a Monday, we gave Mrs. W. a clear liquid diet and 1 gram of neomycin every 4 hours. On Wednesday evening we gave her tap water enemas until they ran clear, and a 250 cc retention enema of neomycin sulfate, which she held for 6 hours. She was now NPO. The surgical resident inserted a central venous pressure line and started intravenous fluids to maintain hydration through the night. Next morning, morphine and atropine were given as preoperative medications.

To remove the bladder, urethra, uterus, and pelvic lymph nodes and create an ileal "loop" to divert the urine outside through a stoma, also newly created, took 7 hours.

Mrs. W. entered the recovery room with a temporary plastic bag over the stoma. After 2 hours, she was transferred to the intensive care unit, where the nurse there placed a humidifying mask over her face so that coughing and deep breathing would be easier.

The nurse checked Mrs. W.'s vital signs frequently and her central venous pressure every hour. Initially, her urine, which was pink, had a specific gravity of 1.020. Feeling that she was behind in her fluid needs, the doctor ordered her I.V. flow rate stepped up to 150 cc/hour for 4 hours and 500 cc of Plasmanate to be given over the next 6 hours. Mrs. W.'s urinary output went up to 80 cc/hour and the specific gravity fell to 1.013. Her vital signs and CVP remained stable; her abdominal dressing, dry with no blood or urinary leakage; her stoma, a good bright red with no bleeding; and her appliance, intact with no urine seeping onto the skin. This was all as it should be.

The ICU nurses continued their vigil with Mrs. W., though, because the patient who has just had a cystectomy can often be acutely ill. With the removal of so much tissue including the bladder, the patient can easily develop surgical shock, cardiac decompensation, or thrombosis.

The nasogastric tube placed during surgery to relieve any pressure on Mrs. W.'s small bowel intestinal anastomosis was draining 250-500 cc of greenish fluid during each 8-hour period. This fluid was replaced with an appropriate I.V. fluid along with her other I.V. fluids.

Despite discomfort from the long abdominal incision, Mrs. W. cooperated when the nurses gave her coughing and deep breathing exercises every hour and helped her turn in bed at least every 2 hours. Every 2 hours also, they gave full range-of-motion exercise to her legs and twice a day removed the surgical stockings she had worn ever since she went to

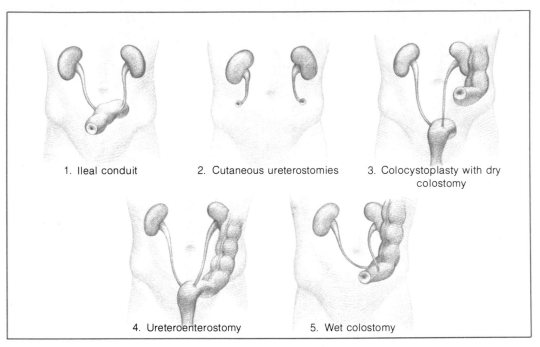

1. Ileal conduit   2. Cutaneous ureterostomies   3. Colocystoplasty with dry colostomy

4. Ureteroenterostomy   5. Wet colostomy

surgery. All these measures were to prevent thrombophlebitis and pulmonary emboli. The latter is a special risk where pelvic tissue is dissected and manipulated.

Kidney function was tested daily through hemoglobin, BUN, and creatinine, and the risk of electrolyte imbalance was offset by daily testing, too. Additional potassium was added to the I.V. fluids.

Mrs. W. remained in ICU for 4 days. She was discharged from that unit to our floor the day her NG tube was removed. Though she had a few bowel sounds, she had not passed flatus; so she was still given nothing by mouth. That evening bowel sounds became very active and she developed explosive diarrhea. The resident attributed it to the ampicillin (Penbritin) she had been receiving since surgery as a prophylaxis against infection. That was stopped now and she was started on diphenoxylate hydrochloride (Lomotil) (Retardin) and a clear liquid diet. Next day, when her fluid intake was adequate and the diarrhea controlled, the I.V. line was removed. A superficial phlebitis had developed at the needle site; hot packs relieved the discomfort.

During Mrs. W.'s initial postoperative period her stoma

remained a healthy red and her urinary appliance stayed intact for several days at a time. On her 12th postoperative day she was fitted with her permanent appliance. Plans were being made for her discharge as soon as she felt able to care for herself.

Shaping the future

Since 71% of all patients who've undergone surgery for localized bladder cancer will survive at least 5 years, your instructions on self-care of the stoma can really shape their future. Will they reject their stoma because they suffer the embarrassment and discomfort of leaking urine, an unpleasant odor, or a bulky pouch? Or will they learn to accept their stoma and gain confidence in their security from accidents?

We gave Mrs. W. the following step-by-step instructions in self-care, as we do with all patients with urinary stomas. When changing appliances for patients in the hospital, you should follow these instructions too. They'll learn self-care more quickly if you establish a firm routine early in their care.

Before removing the appliance, assemble all the necessary equipment: adhesive solvent in a large container and in a small bottle with an eye dropper, cotton balls, skin prep adhesive (in a spray can or as small pledgets wrapped in foil), warm water and cloth, paper tape, and the new appliance. If still using temporary appliances, make sure the opening has been cut to the proper size.

Remove the appliance, using the solvent in the eye dropper to gradually loosen the faceplate (photo 1, next page). Don't use any force when removing the appliance; it can damage the skin. Place a cotton ball over the stoma to collect the urine; remove it when it becomes damp and replace with a dry one.

Carefully remove all adhesive material from the skin using the solvent solution from the larger container. Gently wash the area with warm water to remove the solvent. Don't use soap. Allow the skin to air-dry, changing the cotton over the stoma opening as needed to prevent urine from leaking on the cleansed area.

If the skin under the faceplate is reddened, use a light powdering of Karaya powder to protect the skin and allow healing. More serious skin excoriation will require orders from the doctor or enterostomal therapist.

Spray on adhesive or use the adhesive pledgets to cover an

A host of diversions

The figures on the opposite page show several methods of urinary diversion. In the method most frequently used, the ileal conduit or ileal bladder (Figure 1), the doctor anastomoses the ureters to an isolated ileum segment. He then brings the ileum segment through the abdominal wall to form a stoma. The remaining colon is sutured together and functions normally.

In cutaneous ureterostomies (Figure 2), the doctor leaves the colon intact and brings the ureters to the abdominal surface as stomas. Some doctors prefer this procedure for its simplicity but others dislike it because the patient has constant urine drainage.

In a colocystoplasty, (Figure 3), the doctor divides the sigmoid colon and brings the proximal loop to the abdominal surface to form a dry colostomy. He then closes the distal portion of the sigmoid colon to form a pouch and transplants the ureters into this pouch, sending urine out the rectum. Although this diversion separates urinary and colon functions, it creates one disadvantage: drainage problems and urinary incontinence.

In a ureteroenterostomy (Figure 4) the doctor transplants the ureters into the intestine, and in a wet colostomy (Figure 5) he transplants them into the descending colon, which is then brought through the abdominal wall to form a stoma. These methods gained quite a bit of popularity several years ago. But because they cause a high incidence of renal infection, ureteral obstruction, and hydronephrosis, doctors seldom use them now.

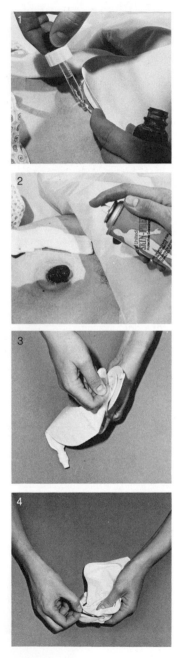

area equal to the size of the faceplate (photo 2). If you're using a reusable faceplate, assemble it by stretching the pouch opening over the rim of the faceplate (photo 3). To keep the pouch in place and prevent leaks, slide a rubber O-ring over the pouch and into the groove in the faceplate rim (photo 4). Take the adhesive off one side of a double-sided adhesive disc and apply the disc to the faceplate (photo 5). You may want to apply a dissolvable stoma guide strip inside the faceplate opening (photo 6). Remove the backing on the adhesive disc and apply the appliance. Be sure to center it over the stoma (photo 7). If the patient is still spending a lot of time lying down, direct the outlet to the side. If he's ambulatory, place the bag so the outlet is toward the leg. Keep the appliance in place with a stoma belt or paper tape (photo 8).

With reusable appliances, clean the adhesive from the faceplate and rinse it with cold water. Soak the bag and faceplate for several hours in a solution of cold water with 1 tablespoon of vinegar added to every quart of water; soaking will decrease the urinary odor.

Far from ideal
By the time she was discharged, Mrs. W. was caring well for her stoma and adjusting psychologically. From almost everyone's standpoint, she was an ideal patient. Except for her diarrhea and superficial phlebitis, her postoperative course was quite smooth. But this isn't always the case. Only by observing a patient closely and handling situations promptly can you detect or help the doctor handle complications.

• *Necrosis of the stoma.* The first sign of necrosis is a dark discoloration of the stoma. You should report this immediately to the urologist so he can examine the stoma with a cystoscope. Necrosis may stem from thickness of the abdominal wall inhibiting blood flow to the surface, a poor fit of the appliance causing leakage, or the skin's reaction to the appliance.

As time goes by, the stoma may become increasingly necrotic and partly separate at the skin edges. Despite your efforts at skin care, skin around the stoma and in the groin may become excoriated. The doctor may order light treatments to the excoriated areas, followed by an application of nystatin (Mycolog powder and Mycostatin spray). For your part, make sure the collection bag fits properly around the stoma — snugly enough to minimize skin excoriation but loosely enough to avoid constriction. You might also use a special skin cement, such as Skin Bond, to firmly hold the appliance.

• *Deep vessel phlebitis.* The first symptoms of this complication may be severe leg and groin pain. Be sure to ask your patient if he has any pain, since he may neglect to mention it, either because he doesn't want to complain or because he fears it will mean additional treatments. The usual treatment for thrombosis and phlebitis starts with I.V. anticoagulation with heparin. After pain has subsided, start the patient on sodium warfarin (Coumadin) and fit him with thigh-length antiembolism stockings.

• *Stomal stenosis.* Sometimes edema of the stomal opening can cause urinary tract infections, often characterized by shaking chills and fever as high as 105°. The chills and fever follow retention of urine because the stomal opening is virtually closed, as both X-rays and your own observation of the stoma may reveal. Pyelonephritis can result from urine backing up into the kidneys. Treatment for this complication includes a prolonged course of antibiotic therapy to eradicate the infection followed by surgical revision of the stoma.

• *Ureteral obstruction.* Another occasional complication is mechanical obstruction of the ureter caused by calculi or calcium deposits, or mechanical obstruction. (Be particularly watchful for it in patients who drink a lot of milk, as those with difficulty eating often do.) Ureteral obstruction can cause uremia, characterized by nausea, vomiting, perspiration, and elevation in blood pressure, BUN, creatinine, and potassium. If unchecked it can lead to coma and convulsions.

The treatment for ureteral obstruction caused by calculi or calcium deposits is restriction of milk and other protein, usually to 40 grams per day. The treatment for mechanical obstruction is surgical reconstruction. Check with the dietitian for instructions.

• *Extensive metastasis.* Some patients first appear with a highly invasive and aggressive anaplastic lesion that scarcely responds to therapy; these tumors usually have also metastasized by the time they're discovered. Following surgery, such a patient may be given chemotherapy, usually 5-fluorouracil (5-FU), doxorubicin hydrochloride (Adriamycin), or mitomycin C (Mutamycin). Their effect on longevity

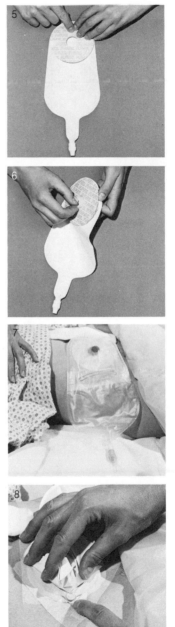

can't yet be evaluated. Some patients receive radioisotope implants for a short time. These can cause cystitis and proctitis, which must be treated by fluids, analgesics, sedatives, antispasmodics, and stool softeners. Watch for symptoms: frequent, painful urination; rectal pain; frequent urge to defecate but inability to pass feces; mucus, blood, or pus in feces. Also save all drainage from a patient treated with radioisotopes so it can be monitored.

Altered body image

By physical measures such as those I've described, you can restore the patient to optimum health and function. But with these patients, your physical care is only as good as your emotional support. For, like patients with colostomies, patients with urinary stomas need lots of help to adapt to their altered body. Chapters 9 and 3 explain how you can give patients emotional support through this trying time. You also should explain the effects of surgery on sexual function.

Though women lose their uterus to the surgery, most are past the childbearing age. For men, though, the crisis is usually more severe. A man may be devastated to learn he will be impotent after the operation. Some may consistently refuse the surgery even though they know the consequences. One of our patients, Mr. M., tried to bargain with the surgeon to do only part of the operation "so I can still be a man."

Not all male patients are like Mr. M. Others have the surgery and will freely discuss their fears about losing their sexual function. You should talk with the patients and their wives, focusing on the independence to be regained, including their jobs and projects, and on the love and companionship they can still share in their marriages. One man who had his bladder removed because of a severe traumatic injury told me, "You know, if sex were all my marriage was about, it would be pretty sad." This is what you should try to help all patients see.

By helping patients adjust emotionally to the changes in their sexual function and appearance, you'll bring them several steps closer to a full, productive life. Of course, you can't take them all the way there; only daily self-care, a healthy attitude, and time can do that. But your psychological support, combined with your good physical care and detailed patient education, will make the trip much easier.

SKILLCHECK 4

1. Wilma Olson, a 62-year-old obese farm woman, had a radical vulvectomy seven days ago. Three days postop, she was ambulating in her room with two nurses assisting and by the fifth day she was helping them irrigate her perineal wound during Sitz baths. Today, you notice a foul odor when you change her bed pad. Does Mrs. Olson have a problem?

2. W. T. (Buzz) Bradley is a husky, 55-year-old divorced football coach who has just undergone a radical prostatectomy and orchiectomy for cancer of the prostate. He will receive diethystilbestrol before he leaves the hospital and later return for radiation. His history shows that he has been sexually active and you suspect he may be profoundly disturbed by the body changes and physical symptoms that will occur from his treatment. What can you do to help him?

3. Margaret Pulaski, a 49-year-old mother of four, was admitted to the hospital with endometrial cancer. She was treated with external radiation, then a radical hysterectomy. Three days postop, she had solid food for breakfast, but immediately afterward she complained of nausea and was given Compazine 5 mg. During the next hour, she complained of abdominal pain and vomited a greenish-looking material. How would you assess her problem?

4. Frank Hines is a 62-year-old printer, who has been inking plates for 25 years. Possibly because of his prolonged exposure to industrial carcinogens, he developed cancer of the bladder and had the tumor removed by transurethral resection. No evidence of local invasion was found at that time, but Mr. Hines was told to return four months postop for a cystoscopy. Now he calls and says he doesn't need to come in, because he has no symptoms. What do you tell him?

5. Sixty-five-year-old Carter Stone lives with his son and daughter-in-law in a small bungalow in the suburbs. After a transurethral resection for cancer of the prostate, he is recovering well and expects to be discharged from the hospital within a few days. His catheter has been removed and he is voiding every two or three hours with gradually decreasing dysuria. But he appears to be very anxious about his voiding difficulties. What can you teach Mr. Stone to reduce his anxiety and prepare him for his return home?

6. Eric Simmons, a 62 year old with an ileal conduit, comes to the emergency room complaining of rectal bleeding. Six months earlier, he had a bladder resection for cancer of the bladder and the surgery was preceded by radiation. The physician in the emergency room diagnoses his bleeding as proctitis. However, Mr. Simmons is extremely depressed and worried that the cancer has spread. How can you help?

7. Sally McConnell, a nervous 39-year-old advertising copywriter, had her Foley catheter removed at 8 a.m., two days after a total hysterectomy. At 11:30 a.m., shortly before she was to receive her pain medication, she complained of severe discomfort in her lower abdomen. She is distressed and near tears. What do you do?

8. Albert Marsella is a 67-year-old retired house painter who is two days postop a transurethral resection and orchiectomy for prostate cancer. He has a Foley catheter with continuous 0.9% saline irrigation, yet when you answer his bell, he complains that he needs to urinate and "move his bowels." What do you do now?

9. Yesterday, Leo Busczek, a 62-year-old baker, had a cystectomy with a urinary diversion via an ileal conduit. He has a temporary ileostomy bag over the stoma for urine collection until he can be fitted with a permanent appliance. This morning, he complains of lower abdominal pain. When you check his output, you find that it has decreased over the past three hours. What other assessments would you make?

(Answers on page 180)

CARING FOR PATIENTS WITH OTHER CANCERS

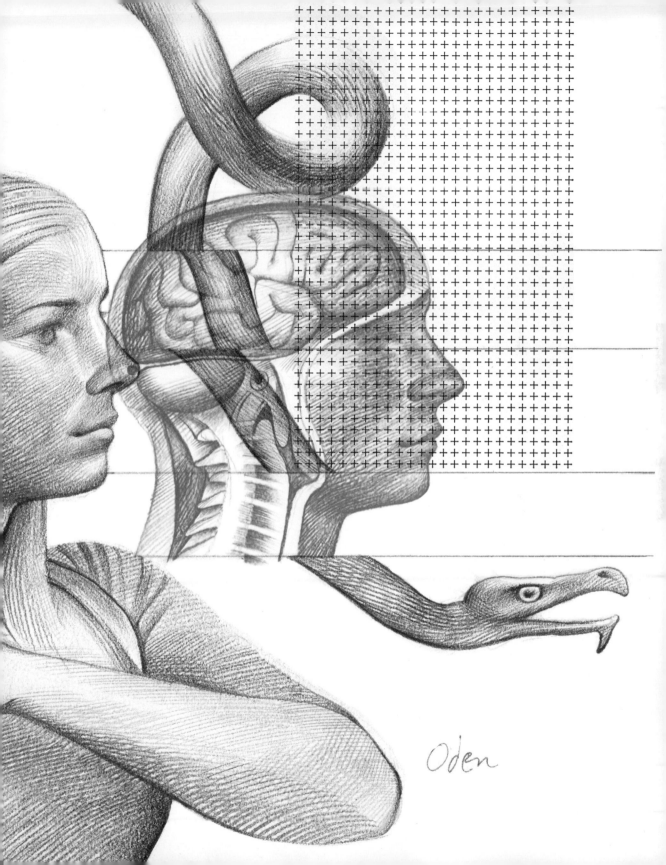

Oden

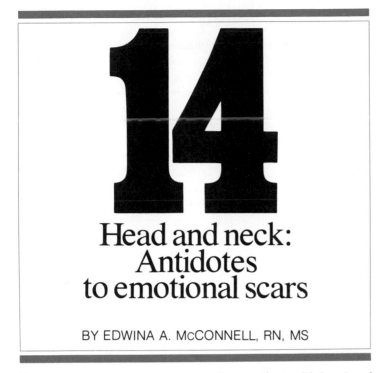

14

Head and neck:
Antidotes
to emotional scars

BY EDWINA A. McCONNELL, RN, MS

SOONER OR LATER, you may care for a patient with head and neck cancer. Will you know how to prepare him for the disfiguring surgery that may be part of his treatment? Will you know what to say to his family? What about postop problems: Can you recognize and deal with a postop carotid "blowout," a dangerous pharyngeal fistula, flap slough, or chyle leak? You'll find nursing care for these and other problems in this chapter. The skills you learn in the following paragraphs may save your patient's life.

Cutting out the killer
Suppose you have a patient like Mr. J., who was first admitted to the hospital with cancer of the right jaw. The cancer was excised locally, and Mr. J. received radiotherapy to the primary area and nearby neck. Two years later, he returned with cancer at the base of his tongue. The surgeon did a complete resection of the right mandible, a resection of the right base of the tongue, and a right-sided radical neck dissection. This was done even though the lymph nodes and the area surrounding the cancer looked normal.

Why such extensive surgery with no palpable lymph nodes?

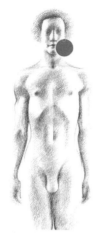

**Pathophysiology:
What you should know**
Of head and neck cancers 35%
occur in the oral cavity, 25% in the
larynx, 14% in the pharynx and
thyroid, and 12% in the lips with
the lower lip being affected
approximately ten times more
often than the upper. The earliest
signs are blisters, scabs, and
ulcers that don't heal.

Nearly all of these cancers are
squamous cell carcinomas. The
deadliness increases in sites
closer to the nasopharynx, the
lowest being in the lip and the
highest in the tongue. Oral lesions
take many forms: ulcerative,
exophytic, infiltrating, fissured,
and so on. Oral tumors spread
locally and through the lymphatic
system rather than through the
bloodstream.

Cancers on the true vocal cords
(intrinsic) don't spread as rapidly
as other neck cancers, because
there are no lymph nodes in the
underlying connective tissue.
Other laryngeal cancers
(extrinsic) spread and
metastasize early, however.
That's why treatment for laryngeal
cancer varies so, including
laryngectomy (partial or total),
radiotherapy, or a combination of
both.

Well, head and neck cancers (which may include cancer of the
lip, gums, tongue, palate, mouth mucosa, tonsils, pharynx,
and larynx) sometimes metastasize into the neck's lymphatic
chain before the primary lesion is even discovered. Fewer
patients die from the cancer's recurrence at the primary site
(after treatment) or from another primary lesion, than they do
from the cancer's spread to the lymph system. Most
oropharyngeal cancers grow slowly, but they're quick to
metastasize. The metastatic lesions eventually kill by pressure
on the trachea, esophagus, blood vessels, and cervical nerves.

Radical neck dissection can be part of a composite resection, as Mr. J.'s was, or it can be a procedure in itself. Sometimes, it's combined with chemotherapy or radiotherapy to
control the primary cancer. Unfortunately, radiotherapy may
cause serious postop complications: delayed wound healing,
pharyngeal fistulae, and life-threatening carotid "blowout."

Preop care
The patient about to undergo extensive surgery for head and
neck cancer needs all the compassion, skill, and individualized
attention you can give him. A radical neck dissection can be
very disfiguring, especially when it involves facial surgery, so
your patient will suffer emotionally — and so will his family.
He may lose his voice (if the larynx is removed) and with it his
occupation, in some cases. He'll have fears about his coping
ability, fears about how people will accept him, and fears
about death.

To prepare your patient and his family for what's ahead,
learn all you can about their personalities, needs, values, and
support systems. Listen sympathetically for what the disease
and surgery mean to the patient and his family. What are their
coping mechanisms? Denial, anger, depression, rationaliza-
tion, repression, compensation, regression — or others? (See
Chapter 3 for details on the patient who won't talk about his
illness.)

When you explain to the patient and his family what will
happen during and after surgery, demonstrate the tubes the
patient will have, and discuss why they're necessary. He may
worry about communicating later, if he's to have a permanent
or temporary tracheostomy, so give him a Magic Slate with a
pencil attached or some cards with simple postop needs pictured on them. Assure him that you'll put a sign by the inter-

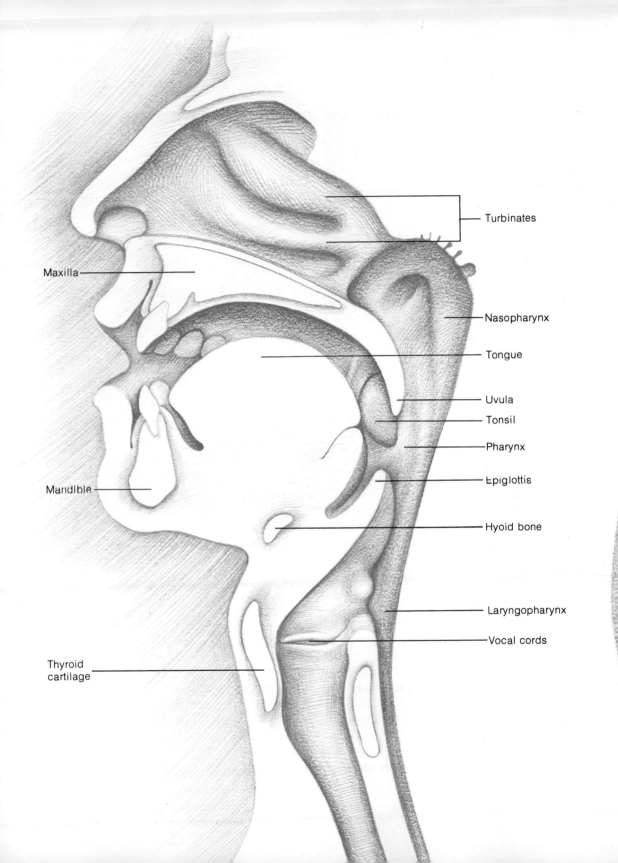

Turbinates

Maxilla

Nasopharynx

Tongue

Uvula

Tonsil

Pharynx

Epiglottis

Mandible

Hyoid bone

Laryngopharynx

Vocal cords

Thyroid
cartilage

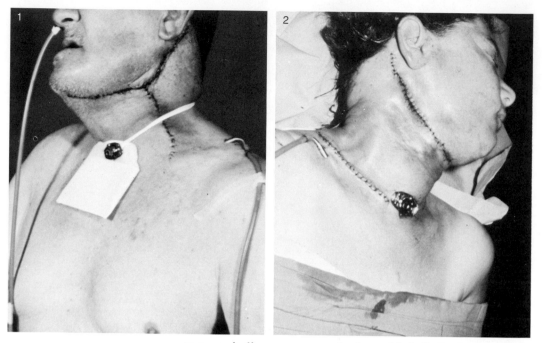

com reminding everyone who hears his bell that he can't talk.

Will your laryngectomy patient lose his voice permanently? A preop visit by a speech therapist may reassure him that he can eventually learn esophageal speech. If the physician approves, you may also arrange for a visit by a rehabilitated laryngectomee through the hospital's social service department or the American Cancer Society. Not every patient reacts favorably to such visits, however, so arrange visits judiciously.

Postop priorities

What are your patient's postop needs? Mr. J. returned from the recovery room with two red Robinson catheters draining his neck wound, a tracheostomy, a nasogastric tube, and an intravenous line. How you care for your patient at this point depends in part on the extensiveness of surgery, the location of the incision, the presence or absence of a tracheostomy, the patient's ability to swallow and talk, and the coping mechanisms of both the patient and his family. Postoperatively, your long-range objective is to help the patient and his family deal with the surgery's aftereffects. Your immediate task: Prevent or treat surgical complications; keep the patient's pain and discomfort to a minimum; and relieve his anxiety as much as possible.

Here's a list of priorities to follow:
- check airway
- elevate head of bed
- interpret vital signs
- measure intake/output
- care for tracheostomy if there is one
- maintain wound suction
- give analgesics as ordered
- give mouth care
- give nasogastric (or pharyngostomy) tube care.

With Mr. J., we checked his trach at once for an open airway. (When there is no tracheostomy, you can check the airway by placing your hand an inch or so from the patient's nose and mouth and evaluating the amount of air blown upon your hand.) Though Mr. J.'s airway was unobstructed, we still watched for signs of air hunger: labored breathing, restlessness, apprehension, and disorientation. A patient can be short of air without appearing cyanotic. On the other hand, if Mr. J.'s face was dusky, that could mean venous congestion from ligation during surgery, rather than poor aeration.

Suppose an obstruction develops? If you can't relieve it by suctioning and removing the inner cannula, call a physician. When the patient has a permanent trach, you can even remove the outer cannula (in an extreme emergency) because the trachea is sutured to skin and the stoma can't collapse. But prevent a respiratory emergency by keeping your patient's tracheobronchial tube free of secretions. Keep it patent with proper suctioning and cleaning; prevent crusts from forming with a humidifier or mist collar. When you replace the inner cannula after cleaning, be careful not to occlude it with the tracheostomy dressing or tape.

Encourage him to turn, cough, and deep breathe — supporting his neck when necessary to keep excessive tension off his sutures. Unless the anesthesiologist orders otherwise, elevate the patient's bed 30° to 45° when he returns from the recovery room. This position (semi-Fowler's) increases lymphatic and venous drainage and venous pressure on the skin flaps, and it makes swallowing easier.

Check the patient's vital signs (using a rectal thermometer),

Which surgery and when

When is a radical neck dissection performed? When a patient has a primary cancer in the neck, has metastasis to the cervical lymph nodes, or has a cancer that must be removed through the lateral neck. It isn't indicated when cancer has spread through the bloodstream (e.g., lymphoma or osteosarcoma of the mandible); when a primary cancer is no longer curable; when there's distant metastases; or when metastatic disease cannot be resected.

A radical neck dissection removes all non-vital neck structures, including cervical lymph nodes on the side with the cancer, some muscles, and afferent and efferent connecting vessels that may contain cancerous tissue.

On the opposite page, Figure 1 shows the postop appearance after dissection. Note the suction catheter, feeding tube, and tracheostomy. Figure 2 shows the postop appearance following dissection for metastasis from a primary tongue cancer. Again you can see the suction catheter and tracheostomy.

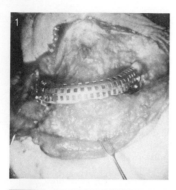

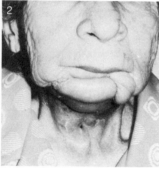

The ravages of surgery
The patient pictured above had a 2 cm squamous cell carcinoma in the midline of the floor of her mouth that had invaded the mandible. Because of the awkward location of the lesion, the physician had to resect the anterior arch of the mandible just to reach the cancer.

During reconstruction the patient had bone grafts taken from her left hip to support her newly created chin and the floor of her mouth. As shown in Figure 1, a metal prosthesis was used to replace the mandible during the insertion of the bone graft. Figure 2 shows the patient's postop appearance after skin grafting and mandible reconstruction.

and measure his intake and output. A change in vital signs suggests several things: edema, throat irritation, pneumonia, hemorrhage, or inadequate wound drainage.

Wound suction is vitally important the first 12 to 18 hours after surgery to drain any collected blood or fluid. Mr. J.'s two red Robinson catheters (inserted below the clavicle) were attached to an Emerson pump at 40 cm water suction. Adequate wound suction not only hastens wound healing and protects skin flap viability, it decreases the likelihood of hematomas, seromas, and air collection in the dead space left by massive tissue resection.

Suppose the catheters clot off? Notify the physician immediately, and if the catheters need to be irrigated, irrigate them using strict aseptic technique. Prep the junction of the catheter and suction tube with an iodine-based antiseptic. Wearing sterile gloves, gently instill a small amount of saline through the catheters. Reconnect the catheters to suction. If they don't clear, repeat the procedure, try again — and (if unsuccessful) call the physician.

Observe the patient's skin flaps for color, possible necrosis (especially around the carotid artery), fluid or air accumulation. The flaps' normal color, the best indicator of adequate blood supply, is usually pale pink. Any sign of bleeding from the wound site or in a necrotic area warns of an impending massive hemorrhage, so call the physician immediately and do not leave the patient unattended.

Because the pain associated with a laryngectomy or radical neck dissection is less severe than that from major abdominal surgery (unless there are complications), mild analgesics should keep your patient comfortable. On the other hand, his emotional pain is probably acute. Listen to his fears and reassure him. Watch for signs of frustration and despair (especially over inability to communicate or altered body image) and give the patient support and encouragement.

Make sure your patient gets frequent, meticulous mouth care, and eventually teach him to irrigate himself to encourage independence. Give mouth care gently to avoid traumatizing exposed or irradiated tissue. If the patient has trouble swallowing, place one end of a wick in the corner of his mouth and the other in an emesis basin. Or supply him with a basin and an ample supply of tissues.

Good nutrition is vital for tissue healing. But normal eating is difficult, if not impossible, for all radical neck surgery patients because of suture lines, swelling, and sometimes the inability to swallow. For these reasons, either a nasogastric tube or cervical pharyngostomy tube is inserted at the time of surgery. At first, the tube is used for intermittent suction to prevent gastric distention and possible aspiration. Later, it's used for feeding.

Some total laryngectomy patients don't have tube feeding, but take food and fluids orally the 2nd postop day. If your patient is one of these, be ready to reassure (and possibly suction) him during the first oral feeding, because he may feel panicky and nervous. (Some hospitals give the patient water with methylene blue to check for fistulae before oral feedings. If a fistula is present, withhold oral feedings till it's healed.)

Pressing postop problems

What complications lie in wait for your patient after head and neck surgery? There are many, depending on the cancer, your patient's physical and mental condition, and the surgery's extensiveness. Other things that may cause difficulties are preoperative radiation, inadequate postoperative care, or faulty surgical technique. (During surgery, the most significant injuries are to vessels: the internal jugular, thoracic duct, subclavian vein, or carotid artery.)

Immediately after surgery, watch for these complications: bleeding into the wound and respiratory distress. Although bleeding into the wound is uncommon, it usually results from inadequate homeostasis. Treat it by aspirating the hematoma or by opening the wound and evacuating it.

In the intermediate postop phase watch for:

• *Pneumonia and atelectasis*. A threat to all surgical patients receiving anesthesia. Monitor chest sounds and watch for for rising temperature. Explain the importance of turning, coughing and deep breathing even if it hurts. If the patient has a trach, keep it suctioned until he can suction it himself.

• *Wound infection*. Avoid this by maintaining adequate negative pressure with drains and suctioning. If you notice necrosis or pus draining from anywhere on the flaps, notify the physician. He may order additional drains and antibiotics.

• *Pharyngeal fistula*. Suspect this major, late complication if saliva leaks from the wound about the 10th postoperative day. Notify the physician. He'll probably discontinue oral feedings, order new drains inserted in the mouth and neck to divert saliva, and prescribe antibiotics.

• *Chyle or lymph leak.* An uncommon, but dangerous complication, in which a fistula on the thoracic duct leaks lymph fluid into the lateral neck wound. Watch for copious drainage (clear, opaque, or milky) from the wound. Notify the physician, who may have to ligate the duct.

• *Flap sloughing.* This occurs in radical neck dissections when the surgeon is unable to save enough blood vessels to adequately nourish the remaining skin flaps. If necrosis is severe enough to invade the carotid artery wall, it can cause a massive hemorrhage.

• *Hemorrhage.* A hemorrhage can occur 8 to 20 days after a wound infection begins, or sooner — because of surgical injury or weakening of the artery from preop radiation. Watch for a bright red stain on the wound's margin or signs of bleeding in necrotic tissue. Notify the physician at once and prepare for an emergency. If the carotid artery ruptures, apply digital pressure with gauze pads, a bath towel, or a sheet. Summon help. Do not leave the patient.

These are some early and intermediate postsurgical complications of extensive head and neck surgery. Others include neural, sensory, and vascular problems resulting from damage to cervical and spinal nerves and muscles. A conscientious exercise program — usually begun on the 10th postop day — is essential to preserve the patient's muscle function.

A positive approach to the future

Proper discharge planning begins when the patient is admitted, and includes teaching the patient and his family home care, involving them, and giving them opportunities to participate. Ensure a smooth transition for the patient from hospital to home by arranging well in advance for a visiting nurse. She can help him adapt the skills he has learned in the hospital to conditions at home, and she can order needed supplies.

Caring for the cancer patient who has undergone head and neck surgery is difficult and requires great skill and compassion. As you've discovered in this chapter, the patient may have numerous preop and postop problems — both physical and psychological. Help him cope with these and support him with a positive attitude — so he can look to the future as a whole person.

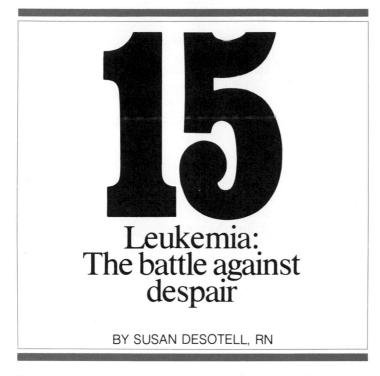

15

Leukemia: The battle against despair

BY SUSAN DESOTELL, RN

OF COURSE YOU'RE AWARE of leukemia's reputation among patients. You've seen the fear and hopelessness the diagnosis engenders in them and their families. But thanks to modern combination therapy, you can counter their despair with honest encouragement. On the other hand, because of its toxicity, modern therapy confronts you with new problems, new challenges.

But first, consider the benefits derived from major advances in drug development and combined agent therapy as well as techniques in supportive therapy, transplantation, and immunotherapy. An encouraging aspect of these advances is that some patients' lives may not only be prolonged but also be made more comfortable and happy by the temporary and possibly permanent remission of symptoms. They offer patients and their families a few more precious months or years together. To those confronted with the loss of a loved one, this reprieve is a priceless gift. It also offers the hope that the patient may benefit from a yet-to-be-discovered cure.

The current treatment, which relies heavily on combinations of potent drugs and radiation directed chiefly at the central nervous system, often leaves leukemia patients nauseous, debilitated, and susceptible to hemorrhage for weeks if not months. Maneuvering a patient through these day-to-day trials is not an easy task in the best of circumstances. But it's especially difficult if your patient is a working woman who felt fine before treatment. Such was the case with a former patient of mine whom I'll call Sarah.

When leukemia strikes

Sarah, just 23 years old, seemed in perfect health until she suddenly developed a flu-like illness with a fever of 102° F., which kept her at home for a few days. She took aspirin until the fever subsided and returned to her secretarial job thinking she had recovered. Still she was bothered by a nagging cough and decided to see her physician.

On examination, he detected rales in the lower bases bilaterally, and a chest X-ray revealed a diffuse lower lobe infiltrate. Probable diagnosis: pneumonia. After additional questioning, Sarah recalled that her last menstrual period lasted abnormally long — 14 days to the best of her recollection — and she had passed clots. This altered the picture and alerted her physician to order a complete blood count to rule out the possibility of something other than pneumonia.

Abnormal bleeding together with an infection are the most common clinical signs of leukemia. Both result from a proliferation of abnormal white blood cells (WBCs), which are too immature to defend against infectious organisms and which crowd out platelets essential for normal blood clotting. Sarah's platelet count had fallen to 40,000 per cu mm (200,000 to 400,000 is normal). Her WBC count was 3500 per cu mm with a pronounced left shift, showing myelocytes and metamyelocytes as well as a small percentage of myeloblasts. (The low WBC count may seem surprising but is common in leukemia patients.)

Sarah's physical examination revealed marked splenomegaly and lymph node enlargement, consistent with leukemia. A bone marrow tap, she was told, would be necessary to confirm the diagnosis.

Despite our efforts to relieve her fears, Sarah was clearly anxious while we were prepping her. Her anxiety increased when she learned that she would experience momentary discomfort as the fluid was being withdrawn. We gave her diazepam (Valium) I.M. before draping and cleansing the

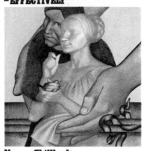
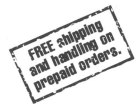
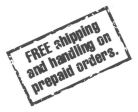
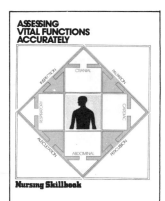
PLEASE DETACH THIS STUB BEFORE MAILING

FIRST CLASS
PERMIT NO. 1903
HICKSVILLE, N.Y

BUSINESS REPLY MAIL
No Postage Stamp Necessary if Mailed in the United States

Postage will be paid by:

Nursing Skillbook

The Skillbook Company
6 Commercial St.
Hicksville, N.Y. 11801

THE TYPES OF LEUKEMIA					
GENERAL CLASS	SUBCLASS	CELL	HISTOCHEMISTRY OR OTHER FEATURES	CLINICAL FEATURES	PROGNOSIS
Acute leukemia	Acute lymphatic (ALL)	T or B type	Sudan black and PAS +	children (0-15 years) lymphadenopathy response to therapy 95%	median 13 mo.
	Acute myeloblastic (AML)	myeloblast	peroxidase +	adults (15-75 years) response to therapy 50%	median 10-12 mo.
	Acute monocytic (AMoL)	monocyte	muramidase +	—	6 wks. to 3 mo.
	Acute myelomonocytic (AMMoL)	—	mixed features morphologically	—	1 to 2 years
	Acute stem cell or undifferentiated leukemia (AUL)	stem cell	no morphologic differentiation	—	very poor
Chronic leukemia	myelogenous (CML)	myelogenous	pH chromosome absent LAP	splenomegaly	median 3 years
	lymphatic (CLL)	B type	immunoglobulin or surface markers	lymphadenopathy	median 5 years

Leukemia: Which type is it?

Although thought of primarily as a childhood disease, leukemia strikes approximately 18,500 adults and 2,500 children a year. A brief look at Table 1 will give you some idea of what's involved in classifying leukemia.

The specific type of leukemia depends entirely on the type of immature WBC that predominates in the peripheral blood. Immature polymorphonuclear leukocytes (polys) are called myeloblasts, and their lymphatic counterparts are lymphoblasts. In most cases, the lymphocytic leukemias can be held in check with chemotherapy and radiation far longer than the myeloblastic types, which generally carry a poor prognosis.

There is also a chronic form of leukemia for each of two predominant cell types. Both chronic forms are adult diseases. Chronic myelogenous leukemia (CML) is characterized by massive splenomegaly with an elevated white blood count. A chromosomal abnormality, referred to as a Philadelphia chromosome, occurs in the white blood cells of patients with CML.

Approximately 80% of patients with CML will convert to acute myeloblastic leukemia (AML) within 2 to 3 years of their initial diagnosis, and almost all will succumb to the disease within 18 months after converting.

Chronic lymphatic leukemia (CLL), on the other hand, almost never converts to the acute type, and the median survival rate exceeds 5 years. Also, no Philadelphia chromosome is present in the WBCs.

As with other forms of leukemia, acute varieties cause large numbers of immature WBCs to accumulate in the marrow and peripheral blood. As the disease progresses, the leukocyte count increases sharply and may reach 50,000 per cu mm.

AML carries a very poor prognosis — in many cases less than 12 months. By contrast, acute lymphatic leukemia (ALL), which is exclusively a childhood disease, has a median survival rate of well over 2 years. Encouragingly, many young leukemics stand a good chance of being cured of their disease.

The key to diagnosis

Abnormal leukemic cells originate in the marrow and, as with other types of cancer, a biopsy of the affected tissue is essential for the diagnosis. Samples of marrow cells are obtained through aspiration or bone marrow biopsy. During aspiration, cellular material suspended in fluid is collected from the marrow cavity of the sternum or the anterior or posterior iliac crest. A marrow biopsy, on the other hand, consists of a solid core of tissue removed from either the anterior or posterior iliac crest. The two techniques are compatible with each other.

If aspiration should fail because the cells are packed too tightly to be withdrawn through a needle, the biopsy can be done at the same site. The entire procedure usually takes no longer than 5 minutes. In many medical centers, the nurse's role in this procedure has expanded from simply answering questions and allaying patients' fears to performing the actual tap.

puncture site on the posterior iliac crest.

Next, the periosteum was infiltrated with a local anesthetic, and the aspirator was inserted into the marrow cavity. Unfortunately, in Sarah's case nothing could be withdrawn through the needle. Such a dry tap indicates that the marrow is choked with a nearly solid mass of cells and little or no surrounding fluid to permit aspiration. In the event of a dry tap, a biopsy will usually produce the desired sample. (One note of caution: Since leukemia patients are often thrombocytopenic, you must apply added pressure to the puncture site to assist clotting.)

Planning treatment

Sarah's marrow biopsy showed the classic picture of acute myelogenous leukemia with a predominance of myeloblasts. With the diagnosis established, the nursing staff began coordinating Sarah's care. At the same time, the hematologist, the oncologist, and the radiotherapist began planning her therapy.

Sarah's physician discussed with her and her family the implications of the disease. He said that the drugs she would receive during the first stage of treatment would combat her leukemic cells, and that if remission could be achieved, the chances of arresting her disease were good. The first phase of treatment, he emphasized, would not only be the most important and the most aggressive, but would also produce some severe side effects.

This conversation left her more upset than reassured. She couldn't understand how she could be so sick when her health had always been excellent until this brief bout with the flu. What exactly was wrong with her blood cells, and how could it really cause her to die? Why should she take these terrible drugs that would make her sicker than she had been?

We told her that she would be hospitalized for the first few weeks of chemotherapy, but that she could learn how to take her drugs on an outpatient basis thereafter. We assured her that a relative could be taught to administer the required daily injection. Other hospitalizations might be required, we told her, but we would help her retain her previous life-style, including her job. A social worker would also be available, we said, to help with any additional problems.

Killing tumor cells

The first phase of treatment, remission induction, relies on drug combinations to kill tumor cells at different stages of their growth cycle. These drugs either kill tumor cells directly (cytocidal) or induce adverse conditions within them so that they are unable to replicate (cytostatic). Several drugs are effective in the treatment of acute leukemia: prednisone, vincristine sulfate, cytosine arabinoside, daunomycin and doxorubicin HCl, 6-mercaptopurine and thioguanine, cyclophosphamide, methotrexate, L-asparaginase, and BCG. Chapters 5 and 6 describes their usual doses and side effects.

Following the bone marrow examination, which served as a guide in establishing the drugs of choice, Sarah was started on cytosine arabinoside (Ara-C) with doxorubicin HCl (Adriamycin). Because Ara-C is rapidly degraded in the blood, it must be given by continuous infusion. Adriamycin was also administered at the infusion site, with care to avoid extravasation since this is an extremely sclerosing substance.

We warned Sarah not to be alarmed if she noticed that her urine was a reddish color, as this is common with Adriamycin use. The drug might also cause her menstrual period to be irregular or even absent, but it would not necessarily alter her fertility.

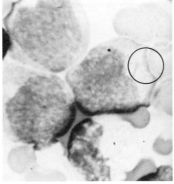

Myeloblasts with Auer body
Myeloblasts are immature leukocytes not normally found in circulating blood. Auer bodies are rods seen in the cytoplasm and are thought to be found exclusively in myelogenous and monocytic leukemia.

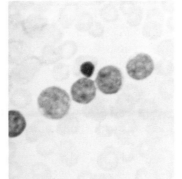

Acute lymphoblastic leukemia
The predominant cells are lymphoblasts with round or oval nuclei that appear "stippled." As compared to the myeloblasts, the chromatin around the edges of the nucleus is more compact suggesting a definite membrane.

As the drugs begin destroying tumor cells, uric acid accumulates in the blood. To avert the possibility of forming renal stones, Sarah was put on allopurinol (Zyloprim) and a high alkaline diet with plenty of fluid to increase uric acid solubility in her urine.

Losing her hair

In fact, much of her therapy was aimed at countering the side effects of chemotherapy described in Chapter 5: abdominal discomfort, anorexia, nausea, vomiting, and alopecia.

Sarah had been alerted to the general nature of expected side effects, but even so, she was not prepared for the impact that chemotherapy had on her body. The sicker she became, the more reassurance and support she required. Most troublesome was nausea and vomiting, which, after many trials, we found could be controlled by high doses of barbiturates and phenothiazines.

Perhaps most emotionally devastating for Sarah was hair loss. We encouraged her to purchase a wig, which, by the way, is covered by most medical insurance plans. But for Sarah, the greatest comfort came from meeting another young patient whose own hair was growing back after chemotherapy. Only then did she believe hers would too.

While we dealt with restoring her confidence in herself and helped her to cope with the side effects of therapy, the hematologist followed her progress with weekly CBCs. Her medication was adjusted in accordance with changes in her blood counts.

Entering phase two

At the end of 4 weeks, a peripheral blood smear showed no immature cells and another bone marrow tap confirmed that she was in remission. Significantly, remission at this stage means that the malignant cells are sensitive to treatment, and that there is a possibility of reconstituting a normal cell population in the marrow, the objective during the next treatment phase.

Phase two, called remission consolidation, combines chemo- and radiotherapies. Methotrexate, vincristine, prednisone, mercaptopurine, and asparaginase are used in various combinations to further reduce the leukemic cell population. Unfortunately, most of these drugs do not cross the blood-brain barrier. Leukemic cells sequestered in the meninges may therefore escape the toxic effects of the drugs and cause central nervous system leukemia, an increasing problem with patients whose lives have been prolonged by chemotherapy. Now, however, meningeal leukemia can be prevented with a combination of intrathecal methotrexate (which is injected into the spinal canal) and radiotherapy to the brain. This dual therapy is chiefly responsible for curing children with acute lymphatic leukemia (ALL).

After several days of radiotherapy, Sarah ran into trouble and had to discontinue treatment. Drugs given to her more than a week earlier caused a severe thrombocytopenia. Her platelet count dropped so precipitously (to 10,000 per cu mm) that we told her not to shave her legs or brush her teeth too vigorously, or do anything that might induce bleeding. We further cautioned her to stay away from alcoholic beverages and aspirin, since both can cause gastrointestinal bleeding.

Additionally, we told her to watch for spontaneous vaginal, rectal, or nasal bleeding, and if such bleeding did occur, that she should, if possible, apply direct pressure and come to the hospital.

The following day she suffered a moderate vaginal hemorrhage and, as instructed, came to the hospital at the first sign of bleeding. Vaginal packing and estrogen treatment were tried, but she developed petechial eruptions and needed 4 units of platelets a day for 7 days before her marrow recovered sufficiently.

Sarah's transfusion was predictable: If there's one thing you can say without fail about leukemia patients, it's that sooner or later they will need a transfusion, and probably more than one.

A depleted population of normal WBCs and nearly total immune suppression (as a result of chemotherapy) leaves leukemia patients susceptible to common bacterial invasion. And a low platelet count makes them vulnerable to hemorrhage from bruises, abrasions, or even normal menses. To help combat infection and hemorrhage, platelet and white blood cell transfusions have become nearly routine. It's a good idea to be on familiar ground when talking about such transfusions because very likely the donor will be a member of the patient's family.

Successful transfusion depends on crossmatching blood products for compatibility. The patient's and donor's specific cell characteristics — ABO types and human leukocyte antigens (HLA) — must be matched as closely as possible. Unmatched blood products trigger an immune reaction causing rejection soon after transfusion.

Matched platelet transfusions enable patients with severe myelosuppression to undergo continuous therapy without the risk of devastating hemorrhage. Since platelets circulate in the blood, they can be obtained by connecting a donor directly to a cell-separator machine, which removes the platelets and promptly returns the other components to the bloodstream. Thus, generous donors can repeatedly give platelets.

Donor-supplied white blood cells are also used for treating active infection in the myelosuppressed patient. Because they don't circulate in as high numbers as platelets, WBCs are more difficult to obtain. Thus, it makes good medical sense to line up prospective donors by getting HLA matching done well in advance.

For the next 10 months after her transfusions, Sarah received intermittent intensive chemotherapy alternating Ara-C and thioguanine with the POMP series (see Chapter 5). At this juncture, when the leukemic cell population was at its lowest, her doctors decided to move on to the next phase, remission maintenance.

The final step
Drug therapy by itself cannot achieve a complete cure because a percentage of leukemic cells remain viable after each drug exposure. Also, prolonged chemotherapy suppresses normal cells to the extent that significant problems such as ulcers may develop.

Immunotherapy overcomes these two drawbacks of long-term chemotherapy.

Sarah seemed a good candidate for BCG (see Chapter 6) because her lymphocytes, although normal by this time in number and distribution, did not respond to antigenic stimulation. Such stimulation was attempted by injecting P.P.D., Monilia, and mumps antigens intradermally, but Sarah failed to develop a sensitivity reaction. If her immune system had been functioning normally, a skin reaction, similar to a P.O.D. "take," would have appeared.

Sarah's lack of immune reactivity was a direct reflection of the impact of chemotherapy on her immune system. Without

BONE MARROW TRANSPLANT: A SECOND CHANCE FOR LIFE

Even though few institutions are performing bone marrow transplants and few patients are undergoing them, they do offer hope for leukemia patients in the future. For nearly half of those undergoing this procedure today, it means another 3 months of life; for about a fifth, it means at least another year — and often more.

Patients eligible for a bone marrow transplant include those with acute lymphocytic leukemia who've had a relapse after treatment or who never achieved remission, those with acute myelogenous leukemia who've had a relapse or have a poor prognosis, and those with chronic myelocytic leukemia that's in the blastic stage. Ineligible patients are those with cardiac disease or renal disease; those who've had maximum radiation treatment to the central nervous system; and those younger than 5 or older than 50. (Those with the best chance for survival are usually in their late 20s or early 30s.)

One more requirement for a bone marrow transplant: a suitable donor, one that matches the patient's ABO and HLA. In most cases, this is a brother or sister, since chances of finding a donor from the general population are almost nonexistent.

How it's done
On the day of the procedure, doctors give the donor a general anesthetic. Then, using needle aspirations, they withdraw 400 to 700 ml of bone marrow from his iliac crests (photo 1). Nurses filter (photo 2) and heparinize the marrow and mix it with culture media for infusion.

Before infusion, nurses give the patient a shampoo and a pHisoHex bath to reduce his body flora; they also apply special

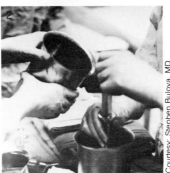

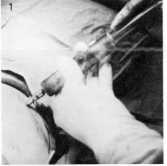

Courtesy: Stephen Bulova, MD

antibiotic ointments to his body orifices. All the leukemic cells in his body are killed by chemotherapy and total irradiation — about 1000 rads administered over 2 to 3 hours. Then he settles in his isolation room and marrow infusion begins.

The patient receives the marrow intravenously (much like any other blood transfusion). Although doctors don't yet know how or why, the new marrow cells reach the bone cavities.

Time will tell
Because the destruction of his WBCs and blood reproductive system renders the patient extremely vulnerable to infection, strict sterile reverse isolation and vigorous antibiotic regimes are essential.

As early as seven days after infusion, when the WBC counts reach their nadir, bone marrow begins to grow again. Until the new marrow functions, however, the patient gets whole blood and granulocyte transfusions daily to avoid hemorrhage and infection. RBC and platelet transfusions may be given daily for 25 days after transplant since their production lags behind that of WBCs. All blood components must be irradiated with 1500 rads before transfusion to kill the lymphocytes that can cause a graft-versus-host reaction. For the first 4 weeks, weekly marrow aspirations and biopsies help confirm a graft "take."

Challenge to success
Several problems may confront the patient in the days to come. He may reject the graft, although doctors can use immuno-suppressants to prevent this from happening. In spite of all precautions, he may suffer a relapse due to leukemic cells resistant to chemotherapy and irradiation. Since his resistance is low, secondary infection may cause leukemia in the new marrow, or the grafted marrow may develop a cancerous growth pattern on its own.

Another complication, unique to marrow transplants, is the graft-versus-host reaction (GVHR): Lymphocytes from the donor's marrow, recognizing the host as foreign, attack the host cells via cell-mediated cytotoxicity. Biopsies show lymphocytes in the skin, liver, and GI tract. A GVHR can be treated with antilymphocyte serum and steroids, but along with infection and heart failure, a GVHR creates a life-threatening situation for the marrow transplant patient.

an active immune system, she was vulnerable to infectious organisms that a competent immune system would have no trouble dealing with.

BCG, we hoped, would provide the needed stimulus to her immune system. The active lymphocytes, in turn, would not only protect her against infection, but would also hunt down and eradicate any lingering leukemic cells. BCG was applied monthly by scarification. Sarah received BCG on eight occasions. Her only problems were flu-like aches with a slight fever easily relieved by acetaminophen (Tylenol) after each treatment.

A year and a half after diagnosis, all treatment was discontinued. A bone marrow examination and lumbar puncture a month later showed normal results.

Sarah's fight against leukemia may not be over. In some hidden recess of her body, a neoplastic cell may be lurking and may begin to proliferate. But she has every right to be optimistic. A few years ago, patients with acute myeloblastic leukemia had a bleak prognosis. To be sure, most such patients continue to succumb to their disease. Nonetheless, chemotherapy, radiotherapy, and immunotherapy now effectively combat leukemic cells, and with each new advance prospects for curing leukemia improve.

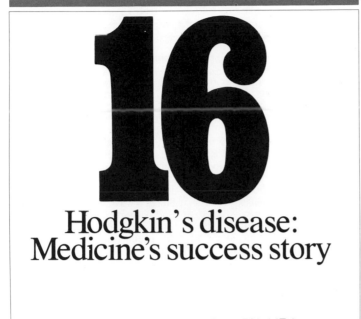

16

Hodgkin's disease:
Medicine's success story

BY JEANNE M. ROGERS, RN, MEd

TO SUSTAIN HOPE is a nurse's prime role. And really, in caring for patients with Hodgkin's disease, sustaining hope is not all that hard to do.

Your task is made easier by one of the great success stories of modern medicine: the story of today's highly effective treatment of Hodgkin's disease.

Oddly enough, many people (including some physicians and nurses) fail to appreciate the implications of this story. Just recently I was talking to a good friend, a top-notch nurse anesthetist. She told me she had assisted that morning in a staging operation on a teenager with Hodgkin's disease. The surgeon had found no evidence that the disease had spread beyond the original site, establishing the stage as IA. My response: "Gee, that's great. You couldn't ask for anything better."

Surprised by my cheerful reaction, she described the atmosphere in the OR during surgery as one of general gloom. The surgeon kept saying, "What a shame for a 16-year-old girl to die of cancer."

Well, there's no longer any justification for such pessimism. With adequate treatment, that youngster will almost surely

WHAT IS HODGKIN'S?

In 1832 Thomas Hodgkin first described a disease characterized by enlarged lymph nodes, an enlarged spleen, and cachexia. Today Hodgkin's disease is categorized as one of four "lymphomas" or primary lymph node diseases. (The other three are lymphosarcoma, giant follicular lymphoblastoma, and reticulum cell sarcoma.) Painless, progressive enlargement of nodal or non-nodal lymphoid tissue characterizes all four conditions.

Although unilateral enlargement of a cervical node generally is the first observable symptom, sometimes the first sign is a bilateral enlargement of several cervical nodes or enlargement of a non-cervical node. The enlarged nodes are usually discrete and movable, varying from the size of a pea to that of an orange (larger nodes are commoner in children).

With Hodgkin's disease in particular, however, a relapsing fever, loss of weight, splenic or hepatic enlargement, or such blood changes as anemia, neutrophilia, or lymphemia may also herald the onset of illness. The presence of Reed-Sternberg cells, absent from other lymphomas, is a presumptive evidence of Hodgkin's disease. But Reed-Sternberg cells have also been reported in patients with infectious mononucleosis, so such cells indicate Hodgkin's disease only if they coexist with one of the four histologic patterns associated with that disease: lymphocyte predominance, mixed cellularity, lymphocyte depletion, and nodular sclerosis. (These patterns have also a prognostic significance: lymphocyte predominance and nodular sclerosis are most common among stage 1 patients, and are generally good prognostic signs. Lymphocyte depletion signifies the worst prognosis.)

Although Hodgkin's disease attracts a lot of public concern, it isn't a common form of malignant cancer, representing only about 1.07% of all cancers in the United States. Public interest in Hodgkin's disease is doubtless related to its frequency among adolescents and young adults. The disease accounts for 14.8% of the cancers afflicting persons 15 to 34 years old. It is almost twice as common among males as among females, and is also more frequently fatal among males. The disease occurs worldwide, among all ages, but rarely in those under 2.

Reed-Sternberg cells from an excised lymph node indicate Hodgkin's disease. Note the large distinct dark nucleoli, a striking feature of these cells.

recover; in fact, her chances of a complete cure are excellent. She will need a few weeks of radiotherapy, which I understand has been scheduled. In addition, she and her family really need adequate emotional support. The responsibility for providing such support rests primarily upon the nursing staff, though others — physicians, radiology technicians, social service personnel — may help in special situations. But in most institutions the burden falls upon the nurses, as they are the only ones in continuous contact with patients, 24 hours a day, 7 days a week.

"What's next?"

When first confronted with the task of providing emotional support for a patient with Hodgkin's disease, some nurses wonder what to say. Ordinarily, you don't begin by talking; you begin by listening. You try to identify the patient's needs and then respond to those needs as they arise.

What the patient needs to know, upon learning that he has Hodgkin's disease, is: What happens next? In most cases, he will not ask what his ultimate fate will be; he understands that no one can predict events in the distant future.

To answer, you will need to understand Hodgkin's disease as it is treated today. A word of warning: A 5-year-old textbook is not a reliable source of such information; therapies and prognoses are changing too rapidly. A more up-to-date source is needed to understand the disease and its current treatment.

Generally, what happens to Hodgkin's patients follows this pattern: The presenting *symptom* is commonly a nonpainful supraclavicular swelling. If *biopsy* establishes Hodgkin's disease, the patient will be referred, often to a special clinic, for *staging* to determine the extent of the disease. In some cases exploratory laparotomy (and perhaps splenectomy) is performed as part of the staging procedure. Depending on the extent of the disease spread, the patient will receive radiotherapy or chemotherapy or both. Patients whose diseases are classified as stage I, II, or IIIA are usually treated with radiotherapy. Chemotherapy is for patients with widespread Hodgkin's disease (stage IIIB and IV) since drugs affect all lymphatic tissues, in contrast to radiotherapy which affects only those within the target area. Combination radiotherapy and chemotherapy treatments often help patients with advanced disease.

Your patient's right to know

Either form of treatment is uncomfortable — and also frightening unless the patient is informed of each new step before it is undertaken. The importance of this was driven home to me by one of my first Hodgkin's patients. He was a man in his mid-forties, at the peak of his professional life. He should have been fully mature, self-controlled, independent. He was not. His body had become a mere object, treated without any meaningful consultation with him. In the year since his disease had been diagnosed, he had learned almost nothing about his condition or its treatment. When I met him, his personality had so deteriorated that he seemed a mere shell. His death was so sad, for he seemed all alone inside.

Right then I decided, no one has a right to do that to a man. It's his body, his life. He may have something important to do or say before he dies. He has a right to know what will happen to him, to consent to the plan.

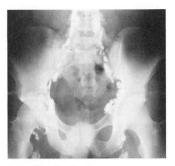

Locating the lesions
The lymphangiogram above reveals enlarged, foamy-appearing lymph nodes in the peritoneal cavity.

In a relatively simple procedure, radiopaque dye solution containing lidocaine is injected intradermally in the first interdigital space in each foot. Within seconds, lymphatic vessels in the feet can be visualized, and one in each foot — usually over the first metatarsal — is catheterized. Over the next hour or 2, ethiodized oil is injected with a pressure injector to fill the lymphatic chain. PA, lateral, and oblique films of the abdomen and chest are taken immediately and 24 hours after injection. These may be repeated in 48 hours. The dye remains in the lymphatic system for several months, and follow-up films may be taken during that time.

Venacavography is generally performed 24 to 48 hours after lymphography. Radiopaque dye is rapidly injected through a catheter in the right femoral vein. PA and lateral films of the abdomen are taken immediately, after 10 minutes, and after 30 minutes. This study permits visualization of the right iliac vein, inferior vena cava, and the ureters upon a background of retroperitoneal lymph nodes filled with a soluble oil.

By comparison, I recall a younger man, about 35 years old, whose disease had also progressed after several remissions. Yet, throughout his therapy, he always understood what was happening and what drug we would try next if the current one failed. We never promised that the new drug would work, nor did we say, "That's a shame but there's nothing more we can do." Until he died, he maintained hope, dignity, and an intact personality. Throughout, he had understood and participated in treatment decisions. He had been a mature partner in the treatment process.

Minimal hospitalization

Fortunately, we see fewer and fewer deaths from Hodgkin's disease. Most patients, we expect, will live, with full health restored. Such patients also need emotional support as they face weeks of therapy, some of it unpleasant. If they can lead near-normal lives during therapy, they will be happier.

I'm thinking of a 20-year-old construction worker from Scranton, a city of 100,000 in northeastern Pennsylvania. Upon discovering a lump in his neck, he recognized its potential seriousness, for his father had major surgery for neck cancer (not Hodgkin's disease) several years earlier. When his doctor diagnosed Hodgkin's disease, the young man insisted on seeking care at a specialized clinic, even though it meant traveling 140 miles to The American Oncologic Hospital in Philadelphia.

When I first saw him he was attempting to cope with several problems: He was worried about the hospital cost; he did not want to burden his family financially while they were attempting to cope with expenses incurred during his father's illness. He missed the emotional support he might have received in his home environment. (I could understand his feeling of unaccustomed isolation, for I too grew up in the Scranton area, where most people live and die within a few miles of where they were born.)

When staging was complete, we had good news for this patient: His disease had not progressed beyond the original site (stage I). We explained that he would require 6 weeks of radiotherapy, but that he could expect to return home and to his old job, fully recovered. Since the actual therapy would require only about 1 hour a day, 5 days a week, we arranged for him to live at the nearby home of one of the hospital volun-

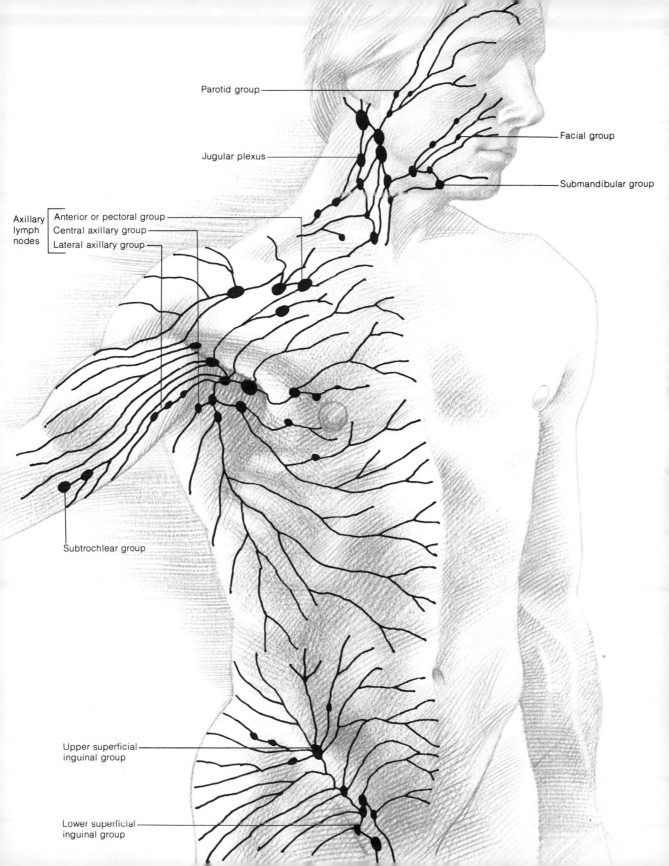

Parotid group

Facial group

Jugular plexus

Submandibular group

Axillary lymph nodes

Anterior or pectoral group
Central axillary group
Lateral axillary group

Subtrochlear group

Upper superficial inguinal group

Lower superficial inguinal group

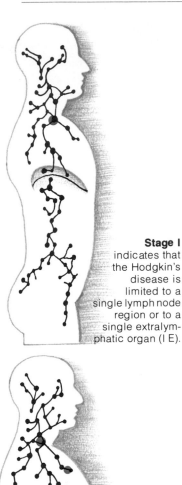

Stage I
indicates that
the Hodgkin's
disease is
limited to a
single lymph node
region or to a
single extralym-
phatic organ (I E).

Stage II
indicates the
disease in two
or more nodes
on the same
side of the
diaphragm:
involvement of
an extralym-
phatic organ
and one or more
node regions (II E)
or of the
spleen (II S).

teers. Thus, he was able to reduce expenses and live in a home atmosphere while obtaining specialized care not available in his own community.

Not every patient can receive radiotherapy as an outpatient, of course. Those who remain hospitalized present a nursing challenge. Treatments take less than a hour a day, leaving the patient with time on his hands. Planned activities — card games, books, arts and crafts, passes outside the hospital — can relieve the tedium. In fact, the value of continued work during treatment is well worth the scheduling problems it presents to the radiology department. It not only fills the hours, but it eases the patient's financial burden and lets him hold on to his job, an important consideration in these days of economic uncertainty.

The emphasis on leading a near-normal life is particularly important for adolescents with Hodgkin's disease. I well remember a high-school junior who worked with us as a candy striper and had recently been accepted into the nursing assistant program at our hospital when she presented with Hodgkin's disease. We delayed therapy a few days so as not to interfere with her junior prom, then scheduled her treatments after 3 p.m. so that she could remain in school, and allowed her to enter the nursing assistant program during the summer recess. Inexplicably this girl, who had become a special favorite of the hospital staff, progressed within 6 months from stage II to stage IV disease and expired following respiratory arrest. The shock to the nursing and medical staffs would be hard to describe, yet our personal involvement (many of us attended her funeral) served a useful purpose: We were able to render emotional support to the girl's family, particularly her mother who still maintains a close relationship with the hospital staff.

Radiotherapy's troublesome side effects
In each of the cases cited, the patient suffered toxic reactions to radiotherapy, yet in no case were these reactions disabling. Recent reports on Hodgkin's disease in the nursing literature describing frightful reactions to radiotherapy are decidedly atypical. In my experience, such extreme reactions are very rare.

This doesn't mean that a patient won't experience highly uncomfortable reactions; indeed, he should be warned to expect them. To fail to provide such a warning would so lessen your credibility with the patient that he might question your optimism about the therapy. You can, however, remind him repeatedly that his discomfort is temporary.

What other adverse side effects can a patient expect from radiotherapy? Gastrointestinal disturbances — anorexia, nausea, vomiting, and diarrhea — because the gastrointestinal mucosa is especially radiosensitive. Fatigue, occasional pain, mild skin reactions, hematuria, stomatitis, and dental decay may also occur. If blood cell and platelet levels fall, there's the chance of anemia and infection. (See Chapter 4 for details on how to combat these complications.)

Since the peak incidence of Hodgkin's disease is between ages 20 and 30, most patients undergoing radiotherapy are concerned about the risk of sterility. Admittedly, the risk of temporary or permanent sterility does exist despite shielding of gonads, surgical repositioning of the ovaries (oophoropexy), and other precautions.

Complications with chemotherapy

What about chemotherapy? Some patients (and their families) still think that antineoplastics can only palliate Hodgkin's disease. This is not necessarily true; chemotherapy may cure. Even if it does not, it does offer the patient the possibility of prolonged productive life, intermittently free from symptoms. Moreover, chemotherapy for Hodgkin's disease is regularly given on an outpatient basis, permitting many patients a reasonably normal life during therapy.

Dozens of chemotherapeutic drugs are being used to treat Hodgkin's disease, alone or in combinations. One of the most effective and commonly used combinations is termed M.O.P.P. protocol. It consists of mechlorethamine (nitrogen mustard), vincristine (Oncovin), procarbazine and prednisone. Drugs are given P.O., I.M., or I.V. push as well as by continuous I.V. infusion over hours or days (see Chapter 5).

Antineoplastic drugs are meant to destroy malignant cells, but they also affect rapidly dividing normal cells, such as hematopoietic cells of the bone marrow, cells of the gastrointestinal epithelium, and cells of the hair follicles. Because of this, a patient may experience many troublesome side effects during chemotherapy. Watch and prepare him for possible gastrointestinal disturbances, alopecia, bone marrow depression, stomatitis, and even pain. A substantial loss of white

Stage III indicates the disease on both sides of the diaphragm: accompanied by involvement of the spleen (III S) or of an extralymphatic organ (III E), or both (III SE).

Stage IV indicates diffuse or disseminated involvement of one of more extralymphatic organs or tissues, with or without associated lymph node involvement.

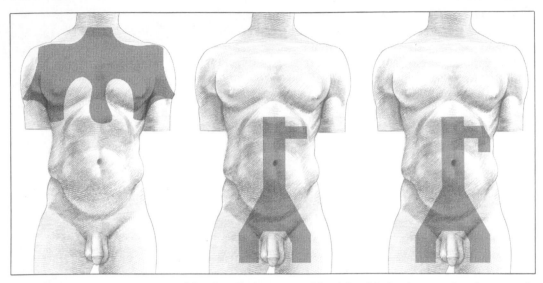

Making mantles for Hodgkin's
Aggressive radiotherapy, given over 8 to 12 weeks, can cure Hodgkin's disease. Cobalt machines are used, but the linear accelerator is preferred. Radiation fields are carefully mapped and therapy is usually given first to the mantle field above the diaphragm and then, if required, to an inverted-Y field below the diaphragm.

Above left is a representation of the mantle field. Note the protection offered the heads of the humeri, the larynx, and the lung fields. The drawing in the center shows the inverted-Y field used in patients who have had splenectomy. Note the extension over the splenic pedicle, and the protection offered the liver and kidneys. At the right is an inverted-Y which includes the spleen.

blood cells increases his risk of infection, and a decrease in platelets may cause oral or nasal bleeding, ecchymosis, petechiae, hematuria, or melena. (For details on how to care for patients with these complications, read Chapter 5.)

Specific drugs can cause special side effects. Neuropathy is a specific side effect of vincristine, causing generalized pain. Fluid retention, hyperglycemia, peptic ulcers, hypertension, and osteoporosis are all possible side effects of corticosteroids. They can also produce temporary mood changes, ranging from euphoria to depression and withdrawal.

An optimistic outlook
No question about it. The side effects of radiotherapy and chemotherapy are frequently unpleasant.

But it would be unfair to end on that note. These therapies are highly effective, in many cases curing this disease that historically has been considered incurable. Even when failing to cure, they produce prolonged remissions, during which patients live comfortable, productive, happy lives. If the patient does not relapse, there are still grounds for hope that therapy can produce yet another remission, possibly permanent.

Hodgkin's disease is one condition for which nurses can realistically hope for excellent response to therapy. And they can honestly encourage patients to hope for the same.

SKILLCHECK 5

1. Fran Bilardo is a 59-year-old chain smoker who had a neck resection for cancer of the left cheek. Two days postop, a check of her vital signs revealed diminished breath sounds and high pitched, crackling rales on her right side. She is reluctant to cough and deep breathe because it hurts her. What complications may be developing and what further assessments would you make?

2. Duane Ferguson, a 42-year-old truck farmer, has just been told by his physician that he has acute myelocytic leukemia. His white blood cell count is 100,000 and his platelet count is 20,000. You know he will be undergoing intensive chemotherapy. What two complications should you watch for particularly and how can you prevent them from occurring?

3. You're trying to help Cynthia Feldman, a busy 24-year-old mother of school-aged twins. She has just been told she has Hodgkin's disease, after biopsy of a nonpainful, supraclavicle lump on her left side. Four weeks earlier, she had noticed a similar lump on her right side, but had done nothing about it. Extreme fatigue finally forced Cynthia to check with her physician, who recommended an immediate biopsy. Now that the diagnosis of Hodgkin's disease is confirmed, Cynthia's physician wants her to remain in the hospital for staging, so he can begin treatment. Cynthia refuses, saying that she must postpone the staging procedure until she has completed her job organizing a PTA fair. What can you do to change her mind?

4. Cynthia Feldman is very upset. Her Hodgkin's disease has just been staged IVB and her physician has recommended that chemotherapy begin immediately. You are discussing her MOPP protocol with her when she begins to cry, saying she knows the doctor lied to her about her stage and prognosis. Her reason for thinking this? She's known other people with Hodgkin's disease who had radiation therapy; she believes that chemotherapy is only palliative, for patients whose disease is far advanced. What would you tell her?

5. Three days have passed since 46-year-old Alfred Sills had a radical neck dissection — preceded by radiation — for invasive laryngeal cancer. You have just cleaned his trach tube, replaced his inner cannula, and are putting back the dressing, taking care not to occlude Mr. Sills' airway. Then you notice heavy pulsations under his skin flap. Is there anything wrong?

6. Julie Sherman is a 29-year-old cashier for a local supermarket. She is currently undergoing induction chemotherapy for acute leukemia and has a white blood count of 1,500. Her temperature is normal. Today, when you're bathing Ms. Sherman, you notice a large, red, fluid-filled sac at the site of a bone marrow aspiration on her posterior iliac crest. How do you assess this finding and what can you do about it?

7. Jason Carlton is scheduled for a radical neck dissection for cancer of the pharnyx. He is a 52-year-old ex-TV program director with a history of alcoholism. Before your admission interview with him, Mr. Carlton discussed the surgery with his physician and appeared to understand it. Now he seems extremely nervous and asks a lot of questions. What can you do to ease his anxiety?

8. You are interviewing Shirley Colburn, a 40-year-old librarian, who has just been admitted to the hospital with leukemia. When you ask her if she has any elimination problems, she confides that she has hemorrhoids and they bother her. How can this complicate the therapy she'll receive and what can you do about it?

9. Joseph Long is a 22-year-old patient who will receive extended mantle radiation treatments for Hodgkin's disease. During your interview with him, you discover that he has trouble eating, which is caused by several decayed teeth. He hasn't been to a dentist for five years, because he's been "too busy." What effect does this have on his treatment plan and what can you do about it?

(Answers on page 181)

SKILLCHECK ANSWERS

ANSWERS TO SKILLCHECK 1 (page 63)

Situation 1 — Jerry Cooper
Obviously, Jerry — as an adolescent — is just beginning to test his independence from his parents. He needs to feel that he is a responsible young adult, and you must take this into account when you work with him. Sit down and discuss this situation personally with him, and find ways that Jerry can be more independent and responsible for his own care. Suggest that he keep a diet diary; also include some of his favorite foods in his diet, if possible. Outline the reasons for proper skin care and explain how complications can slow his treatment. Maintain a relationship of trust with Jerry. Avoid discussing his treatment plan without him present.

Situation 2 — Joseph O'Malley
Find out how Mr. O'Malley feels about going home. He may see the outside world as a threat at this time, because he's not sure how people will react to his disfigurement. He may also be worried about his wife, if she's capable of caring for him, changing his dressings if necessary, and coping with any problems that he might have (dysphagia, swelling, possible infection). Mr. O'Malley may act angry and demanding because he feels like he's lost control over his life. Be reassuring and positive about his return home; enlist the support of his family.

You might have prevented this problem by starting Mr. O'Malley's discharge planning when he was admitted, being consistent with it, and including him in every phase.

Situation 3 — Rita Romano
Without being condescending, find out if Ms. Romano understood that she would go into her menopause after surgery. She may not have realized that the removal of her ovaries would bring it on. Many patients don't understand their body organ functions as well as they should and need a more complete explanation (with charts and diagrams) of surgical procedures. Another possibility is that Ms. Romano understood the function of her ovaries, but was not able to deal with the reality of the situation until that moment.

Ask Ms. Romano what she's heard about menopause from her friends and relatives and try to clear up any misconceptions. Encourage her to ask her physician about it the next morning and remind her that hormonal replacement therapy is available.

Situation 4 — Mary Lou Whitney
Ask Ms. Whitney to return to her room and examine her femoral lymph nodes to see if they're enlarged. A patient receiving BCG injections may develop enlargement and pain in the lymph nodes that drain the injection site. (Usually these nodes are below the injection site. But in this case they would be the femoral, rather than popliteal, nodes.) The swelling may resemble metastases and the physician will have to biopsy the lesion to distinguish the difference.

Check Ms. Whitney for other symptoms. Does she have a fever, chills, or any localized abscesses? Report your findings to the physician. These symptoms may be side effects of the BCG injections and he may put Ms. Whitney on antihistamines and acetaminophen, if he hasn't already. When these symptoms persist, the physician may order isoniazid (INH) 300 mg daily.

Ms. Whitney may also become jaundiced from the BCG, because it has a slight toxic effect on the liver and may elevate the SGOT level. Report jaundice to the physician at once.

Situation 5 — Sara Burke
Sara's anorexia and vomiting is probably caused by her chemotherapy, and aggravated by her depression. Encourage her to talk to you about it, then arrange a visit from the dietitian so Sara can help plan a menu of foods that she enjoys and can tolerate. Order the food for her, if she doesn't feel like doing it, or ask a family member to take on this responsibility. Make sure Sara's surroundings are pleasant when she's served meals, eliminate any bad odors or sounds, and encourage visitors. If Sara complains that her hot food "smells funny," try uncovering it in the hall. This gives the odors a chance to dissipate before she receives her tray. Give mouth care before every meal to overcome any bad taste which may be interfering with Sara's appetite. Try food seasonings to alter flavors that Sara finds distasteful. Use your ingenuity and enlist the support of Sara's family. Perhaps they'd like to bring some of her favorite foods from home and sit with her while she eats. If it's possible, schedule Sara's I.V. chemotherapy for late in the day, followed by an antiemetic. The drowsiness that accompanies the antiemetic may help her sleep through the worst of her nausea.

Situation 6 — John McGinnis
Yes. High fiber foods will irritate John's irradiated

bowel as treatment progresses, eventually causing diarrhea by further injuring damaged tissue. If he stays on his recommended diet, which is low in bulk, he shouldn't have trouble with the constipation he worries about. However, if constipation does develop and lasts for more than two days, John should call his physician. Keep in mind that John is stubborn and may not be willing to change his eating habits. To assure that he does, call his sister and ask for her cooperation. Look into other community resources, such as the Visiting Nurse Association, that might be helpful.

Situation 7 — Frank Calder
Explain the problem to Mr. Calder and reassure him that you will find a way to reduce his pain. Mouth care for stomatitis must always be individualized to fit the patient's needs. With Mr. Calder, it's obvious that his dentures are irritating the aleady damaged buccal tissue and should be removed to prevent bleeding and further pain. Using a lavage bag and a soft rubber catheter, irrigate Mr. Calder's mouth with a solution of hydrogen peroxide and saline. Hang the bag on an I.V. pole, so you can adjust the pressure and flow by raising and lowering the bag. Because Mr. Calder has difficulty expectorating, keep suction ready at all times, using a Yankauer or tonsil tip. Remember to check Mr. Calder's diet before he returns home. He may need an adjustment in his nutritional intake because he will not be wearing his dentures for awhile.

Situation 8 — Betsy Seeger
Start by talking to Betsy personally. Explain that she will lose her hair and that there is no way to prevent it. Encourage her to express her feelings about this, but at the same time stay positive about ways she can keep from "feeling different." With her parents present, discuss the possibility of a wig for Betsy so she can continue going to school without fear of ridicule. Outline the proper care for her scalp, which will be more vulnerable when it loses its protective hair covering. It should be washed as often as needed with baby shampoo and kept dry, then given a thin coating of baby oil if there's a dry skin reaction. If there's a wet reaction, which may occur around the ears, Betsy's scalp should be left uncovered.

To expose her scalp to air as much as possible, Betsy should wear her wig as little as possible at home, relying instead on a cotton scarf in the summer and a woolen stocking cap over the scarf in the winter. If her scalp is always covered, it will perspire, irritating the treated area.

ANSWERS TO SKILLCHECK 2 (page 91)

Situation 1 — Rachel James
By maintaining total independence and approaching her cancer intellectually, Mrs. James may be denying her true feelings. She may also injure herself physically by fracturing her hip or vertebrae, if she continues her present activities. Discuss this possibility with Mrs. James' physician, her husband, and the rest of the clinic staff. Some one whom Mrs. James respects intellectually should warn her about the risks she's taking and offer alternatives.

Keep in mind, though, that Mrs. James has a right to cope with her cancer any way she chooses. She may want to go through the process of dying just as she has lived, and you must allow this. Encourage her to talk about her feelings, but if she doesn't express them, don't push her by prolonging the conversation. You cannot measure the harm cancer has done to Mrs. James, unless you know exactly how she has coped with problems in the past.

Situation 2 — Evan Davis
Ask Mr. Davis to tell you the color and consistency of his sputum. Is it thick and blood-streaked, or is he expectorating blood? Ask if he has a fever, if he feels unusually tired, if he's lost any weight or lost his appetite. The change in his cough, along with the increased frequency of respiratory infections, suggests lung cancer, among other possibilities.

Explain that since he has had 3 respiratory infections, the doctor should examine him before reordering medication. Then check with the physician to see if he wants Mr. Davis to have an X-ray before his appointment.

Situation 3 — Gayle Kaufmann
Turn Ms. Kaufmann onto her back immediately and check for a leak in the chest tube system. Chances are that she has developed a pneumothorax characterized by dyspnea, cyanosis, pain, and profuse sweating. Check all connections for leaks or tube perforations; if one of the chest tubes has slipped out of position, apply a sterile pressure dressing and call the physician to reinsert the tube. Check for breath sounds in the remaining lobe.

However, if there are no problems in the chest tube system, Ms. Kaufmann may be having another significant cardiopulmonary problem. Check her blood pressure, pulse, and respiration; do an EKG strip if she's on a monitor, and notify the physician immediately.

Situation 4 — Elizabeth Berkowitz
Talk to Mr. Berkowitz and the boys. Find out if they understand why Mrs. Berkowitz is incoherent most of the time and if they are aware of her prognosis. Explain her treatment and assure them that you are doing everything possible to make her comfortable.

Try to arrange an opportunity for individual members of the family to be with Mrs. Berkowitz when she wakes up alert at night. If they want, find ways that they can help with her physical care during the day. Some hospitals have group sessions for families of patients with cancer. If your hospital is one of these, suggest this source of support to Mr. Berkowitz and his sons.

Situation 5 — Russell Lawrence
Ask Mr. Lawrence what his physician has told him. He may have misunderstood why the tube was necessary (to reinflate his lung), and still think he had a pneumonectomy. Or perhaps he only heard part of what the physician said about the surgery, because he wasn't listening or was anxious about his prognosis. Whatever you suspect, notify his physician immediately. He may want to talk to Mr. Lawrence again.

Situation 6 — Tillie Ritter
Without a prosthesis to balance her remaining large breast, Miss Ritter may have trouble walking safely and maintaining her erect posture. Improper balance also may aggravate the arthritis in her back. Her clothes won't fit properly and this will alter her appearance, making it difficult for her to be active socially.

Despite her casual attitude, Miss Ritter may not be as carefree about her condition as she would like you to believe. Instead, she may be anxious and afraid of disability. Encourage her to talk about it. Then stimulate her interest in her social activities by reminding her of her friends. Reassure her that she can "go on as before," with the help of a prosthesis—if she wants one.

ANSWERS TO SKILLCHECK 3 (page 117)

Situation 1 — Mrs. Shapiro
Contact Mrs. Shapiro, or have a Visiting Nurse call on her. Her increased use of perfume and air fresheners suggests that she's preoccupied with colostomy odor. She's forgotten how to use the appliance deodorant or alter her diet to control odor.

Check Mrs. Shapiro's irrigation procedure. She may not be irrigating properly, which may cause irregularity and constant fecal drainage. If she's bothered by gas being expelled from her stoma, suggest that she muffle the sound by folding her arms and gently pressing against the stoma. Urge her to avoid gas-producing foods, which contribute to this problem.

Find out why Mrs. Shapiro doesn't want to get dressed and leave the house. She may worry that her colostomy bag will show under her clothes and attract attention. If the physician wants Mrs. Shapiro to visit with a female ostomate, call the United Ostomy Association and arrange a visit. With support from a rehabilitated ostomate, Mrs. Shapiro may gain the strength she needs to rebuild her self image.

Situation 2 — Sheila Katz
Check Mrs. Katz' calves for tenderness, localized heat, and swelling. Measure her calf, if you have any ques-

tion about a change in size. Check for Homans' sign by dorsiflexing her foot and asking her if she feels pain. Suspect thrombophlebitis if these symptoms exist. Check for tachycardia. Notify the physician of your findings.

Situation 3 — Red Taggart
Continue to give Mr. Taggart frequent mouth care. A nasogastric tube in place for more than 12 hours may cause sore throat, dry mouth, hoarseness, earache, sore nose, and dry lips. Provide Mr. Taggart with gargles of warm water or warm saline solution to relieve some of the mouth and throat discomfort. Apply pomade to his lips and nose to soothe sore tissues. Frequent mouth rinsing with saline inhibits saliva production and may encourage dehydration; to prevent this, give Mr. Taggart some cracked ice to suck.

Be alert for symptoms of parotitis: pain, swelling, absence of salivation, and purulent exudate, all of which may occur when a nasogastric tube is left in place for a long time. Chewing gum, if permitted, may help Mr. Taggart prevent obstruction of the parotid ducts.

Situation 4 — Tom Graves
Because Tom works at night, he should irrigate his colostomy about 4 P.M., so it won't interfere with his morning sleeping schedule. To help him start a pattern of bowel regularity, plan his hospital irrigations at this time and explain why you're doing it. Teach Mrs. Graves the irrigation process, also; she may have to care for her husband's colostomy if, for some reason, he can't do it himself.

Situation 5 — Ralph Mott
Check Mr. Mott's condition immediately. Make sure his nasogastric tube is patent and the drainage is not bloody. If the tube is clogged, it will have to be irrigated, but don't do this without an order. Notify the physician at once; do not adjust or remove the tube. Careless handling may injure the patient's suture line or cause abdominal distention.

If Mr. Mott's problem isn't a non-functioning NG tube, it may be bladder distention. Check his Foley catheter (if he has one) to see if it's draining properly. If he has no catheter and his bladder is distended, get an order to catheterize him.

Situation 6 — Albert Johnson
Find out if Mr. Johnson had anything to eat while he was away from home. He may have forgotten or ignored his physician's instructions to eat small meals, especially if he was at a family picnic. His sudden symptoms suggest the dumping syndrome, a late complication of gastrectomy, which may occur within a few minutes after eating. Remind Mr. Johnson and his family that he can avoid these symptoms by eating

smaller meals, resting after eating, and eliminating salt, sugar, and high carbohydrate foods from his diet. Encourage him to drink liquids between, rather than with meals.

Situation 7 — Maria Buckwalter

Reassure Ms. Buckwalter by explaining what has happened, and remove the leaking appliance. Wash the parastomal skin with soap and warm water, then rinse and dry it thoroughly. If the physician has left an order for a topical medication like Kenalog spray, apply the medication to the excoriated area. Call the physician if an order is needed. Then cut a protective barrier of karaya to fit over the stoma and put it in place, making sure the parastomal skin is completely covered. Position a new colostomy appliance over the stoma bud and place a deodorant in the pouch. Notify the physician or enterostomal specialist and watch Ms. Buckwalter carefully for signs of further excoriation.

ANSWERS TO SKILLCHECK 4 (page 145)

Situation 1 — Wilma Olson

Examine Mrs. Olson's incision closely. If you discover purulent drainage oozing from the wound, Mrs. Olson has an infection. Culture the drainage immediately, and notify her physician, who will start her on antibiotics and may order her put in isolation. So Mrs. Olson won't become alarmed by the sudden flurry of activity, explain the situation to her and reassure her. Continue to irrigate the wound with a sterile saline solution, taking care to maintain a strict aseptic technique. Dry the wound by exposing it to the air, but remember to insure Mrs. Olson's privacy when you do this. Remove all foul smelling pads and dressings promptly, especially if she's expecting visitors.

If the wound shows dehiscence from the infection, the physician may open the suture line and drain it. Then he will pack it with sterile gauze soaked in half-strength Betadine.

A patient who is obese may have difficulty cleaning her perineal wound properly, so assist her during Sitz bath irrigations. To prevent further infection, clean Mrs. Olson's wound after each B.M., and remind her not to touch her wound without first washing her hands.

Situation 2 — W. T. (Buzz) Bradley

First, recognize Mr. Bradley's need to mourn and let him express his feelings about his impotence and possible incontinence. Accept the fact that these feelings may swing from despair and hopelessness to unrealistic optimism. Answer Mr. Bradley's questions truthfully, examine your own attitudes to avoid being judgmental, and be positive about the future. Explaining the side effects that Mr. Bradley can expect from DES and radiation treatments will help him prepare for them. Alert him to the possibility of breast enlarge-

ment, beard softening, weight gain, and change in weight distribution from DES therapy. When he begins radiation therapy, warn him that he'll feel fatigued. Extreme fatigue is common for patients undergoing radiation and should be expected. If Mr. Bradley doesn't realize this, he may push himself to exhaustion, then become depressed because he sees it as a sign of physical deterioration. Emphasize the need for regular naps, or if this is impossible, frequent rests. Help Mr. Bradley adjust his schedule so he can rest after treatment.

Situation 3 — Margaret Pulaski

Mrs. Pulaski may have a paralytic ileus secondary to surgery, or possibly an intestinal obstruction precipitated by preop radiation treatments. Find out if she's had a bowel movement. If you see peristaltic waves and her abdomen is distended, suspect an abdominal obstruction. Other symptoms that may indicate obstruction are abdominal pain and frequent, high-pitched peristaltic sounds. (The absence of peristaltic sounds is more likely to mean a paralytic ileus.) Notify the physician. He will probably want Mrs. Pulaski to have abdominal X-rays and be restarted on I.V. therapy.

Situation 4 — Frank Hines

Explain to Mr. Hines that frequent medical follow up is part of good management of bladder cancer, because it allows for early attention to any symptoms that arise.

But find out, if you can, if undergoing the cystoscopy is what's worrying him. This procedure may have been extremely traumatic for him the first time it was done, and he may be afraid to have it repeated. Reassure him that you'll do everything you can to make him comfortable.

Situation 5 — Carter Stone

Start by assuring Mr. Stone that his dysuria and frequency will disappear when his bladder stretches back to its normal capacity. For at least two months, though, he should void whenever he has the urge, to avoid the pressure of a full bladder on his surgical site. Warm tub baths will also help relieve Mr. Stone's discomfort when voiding. So will an increase in fluid intake and the avoidance of spicy foods and alcohol. Mr. Stone can strengthen his weakened sphincter muscle and control dribbling by performing simple perineal exercises: stopping and starting his urinary stream, and tightening and relaxing gluteal muscles. Remind Mr. Stone and his family that he must avoid constipation because straining irritates the surgical site and may cause bleeding. He should continue including bulky foods and plenty of fluids in his diet, as he has done in the hospital. Ask his daughter-in-law to remember this when she plans the family meals. Mr. Stone's physician may also order a stool softener. Tell

Mr. Stone to contact his physician if any problems arise before his next appointment.

Situation 6 — Eric Simmons

Explain the physician's diagnosis to Mr. Simmons. Reassure him that, while metastasis may be a possibility, his bleeding is probably part of the proctitis that is common after bladder irradiation. Because of its proximity to the bladder, the bladder receives radiation and becomes inflamed — causing increased mucosity, diarrhea, rectal bleeding, spasmodic contraction, and pain. These symptoms can be treated easily with an antidiarrheal with or without codeine.

Situation 7 — Sally McConnell

Has Ms. McConnell voided since her catheter was removed? Her discomfort may be caused by urinary retention, which is not uncommon for a patient whose bladder was manipulated during abdominal surgery. Help her to the bathroom, urge her to void, and measure the output. If it's less than 70 cc's, and you notice a distended bladder, you will have to catheterize her residual urine. Depending on the hospital, you may need an order for this. Also check Ms. McConnell's fluid intake. Perhaps it hasn't been enough for her to void naturally. Encourage her to increase her intake and call you again when she has to void.

Situation 8 — Albert Marsella

Check Mr. Marsella's catheter immediately for a decrease in drainage or a change in drainage color. Then check his abdomen for a distended bladder. If his catheter is clogged, causing bladder distention, he may be having a bladder spasm. To relieve it, irrigate the catheter with gentle suction from a Toomey syringe and try to dislodge any clots or tissue shreds. If that doesn't relieve Mr. Marsella's discomfort, notify the physician, who may order an antispasmodic like belladonna and opium suppositories or propanthaline bromide (ProBanthine).

Bladder spasms may also be triggered by the pressure of catheter traction on the surgical site. If traction is initiated, ask the physician for a p.r.n. order for antispasmodics.

Situation 9 — Leo Busczek

Check Mr. Busczek's intake. Lower abdominal pain with decreased output may indicate distention of an isolated segment of the ileum with urine. If allowed to accumulate, the urine may back up into the kidneys or rupture the suture line. Call the physician immediately if you suspect urine accumulation.

Check for fever. If Mr. Busczek's decreased output is from a leak at the ileal conduit anastamosis site or intestinal anastamosis site, he may develop peritonitis, characterized by fever, pain, and a boardlike abdomen. Notify the physician at once if these symptoms occur. Immediate surgical revision with repairs may be necessary.

Check Mr. Busczek's stoma for swelling. Swelling can prevent emptying of the conduit, causing pressure on the anastamosis site. If you notice swelling around the stoma, call the physician.

ANSWERS TO SKILLCHECK 5 (page 175)

Situation 1 — Fran Bilardo

Every patient who receives a general anesthetic runs the risk of developing pneumonia and atelectasis postoperatively. Check Ms. Bilardo's temperature again and report any rise to her physician. Diminished breath sounds, crepitant rales, and an elevated temperature are signs of excess fluid or pus in aveoli. Once again, explain the necessity for coughing and deep breathing to Ms. Bilardo and stay with her while she does it. Try to get her to expectorate. If she brings up any sputum, inspect it for color and consistency; culture it if it's thick or yellow. Listen to her lung and breath sounds. Are they still abnormal? Notify the physician of your findings. Turn Ms. Bilardo frequently.

Situation 2 — Duane Ferguson

Because Mr. Ferguson's white blood cell count is so high, hyperuricemia is one of the first problems you can expect him to have. Hyperuricemia occurs when cytotoxic therapy destroys leukemic cells, leaving uric acid. If the uric acid is allowed to accumulate in Mr. Ferguson's bloodstream, he could develop kidney stones and possibly kidney failure. However, allopurinol administered before and during chemotherapy can inhibit uric acid formation. Monitor Mr. Ferguson's blood uric acid and blood urea nitrogen levels throughout therapy. Speed his excretion of uric acid crystals by keeping him on a high alkaline diet and encouraging him to drink a lot of fluids.

Mr. Ferguson also runs the risk of a cerebral hemorrhage. Hemorrhage can occur in any part of the body when the patient has a low platelet count, but it is most likely in the cerebral blood vessels because of leukostasis. Frequently check Mr. Ferguson's neurological status and look for early signs of hemorrhage: headache, visual disturbances, or disorientation. Notify the physician immediately.

Situation 3 — Cynthia Feldman

Sit down with Cynthia and explain that treatment will begin when staging is completed. Adequate staging allows for careful planning of the best therapeutic approach for her case and offers the best hope for long-term control or cure. Enlist the help of her husband and close relatives. Explain the importance of staging to them, as well as the importance of early treatment. Maybe Cynthia isn't that worried about the PTA fair. Instead, she may be worried about her children, and who will care for them while she is in the hospital. She may also be worried about dying and leaving them without a mother. Discuss these worries with her and with her family, and get the help of the hospital's social service department, if necessary. Help Cynthia work out child care alternatives while she is hospitalized for staging. If possible, secure a pass for Cynthia to go home on a weekend when no staging tests are scheduled.

Situation 4 — Cynthia Feldman

If you weren't present when Cynthia's physician explained her treatment plan to her, contact him and find out exactly what she's been told. Perhaps he'll want to talk to her again. After Cynthia understands why her treatment plan has been chosen, you can work out a way for it to fit with her lifestyle.

Explain the benefits of chemotherapy to Cynthia, but also prepare her for the side effects: alopecia, gastrointestinal disturbances, stomatitis, and mood changes. Before she's discharged, give her the phone number of the hospital's patient-care coordinator, so she can get answers to any questions that she may have later.

Situation 5 — Alfred Sills

Not necessarily. But heavy pulsating of the carotid artery — which may have been damaged during surgery or weakened from radiation — could be the first sign of an impending carotid blowout. Inspect Mr. Sills' wound area for tissue necrosis by gently hyperextending his neck and rotating his head away from the incision. If you see a bright red stain on the wound margin, or any sign of bleeding under the flap (especially in a necrotic area), report it to the physician immediately. If the carotid artery ruptures, apply digital pressure with gauze pads, a bath towel, or a sheet, and summon help. Do not leave the patient.

Situation 6 — Julie Sherman

The fluid-filled sac may be an abscess, teeming with microorganisms. Remember, pus does not form in the absence of granulocytes in a severely leukopenic patient. A patient may have an infection without a typical abscess formation. Place a sterile occlusive dressing over the sac, and adjust Ms. Sherman's position in the bed so there's no pressure on the area. Notify the physician immediately. Infections that remain localized in normal patients may develop into septicemia in leukopenic patients. Inspect your patient's skin daily, because every break in the skin is a potential site for the entry of infectious microorganisms.

Situation 7 — Jason Carlton

Mr. Carlton's reaction could be normal, considering the disfiguring surgery he faces, as well as the cancer. Go over what his physician has told him to make sure he understands everything; listen to his questions and answer him truthfully. Show him ways that he can communicate immediately after his surgery; for example, he can use a pad and pencil. Assure him that there'll be a sign next to his button on the intercom reminding the staff that he can't talk.

But keep in mind that Mr. Carlton is an alcoholic and his increasing nervousness could be a withdrawal symptom. He may need tranquilizers before surgery or he could have DT's. Notify his physician immediately and make sure protective restraints are available, in case Mr. Carlton becomes violent.

Situation 8 — Shirley Colburn

Invasive cancer may cause thrombosis of small vessels throughout the body. When they occur in this area, there is the risk of abscess and infection because of the large number of pathogens. Chemotherapy will depress Ms. Colburn's leukocyte production and she will lose some of her ability to fight infection if it occurs. You can reduce the possibility of abscess and infection by instructing Ms. Colburn in proper perineal care and avoiding trauma to her hemorrhoids. Don't use rectal thermometers, rectal medications, or enemas, unless necessary. Remind Ms. Colburn that she can easily contract a vaginal or bladder infection by improper wiping after bowel movements. Ask Ms. Colburn about her eating habits which may be causing constipation and aggravating her hemorrhoids. Encourage her to drink more fluids and ask the physician if he wants to order a stool softener. Decrease any discomfort she has in the rectal area with Sitz baths, topical anesthetics, and stool softeners.

Situation 9 — Joseph Long

Make arrangements for Mr. Long to have his badly decayed teeth removed before radiation treatments begin. His remaining teeth will have to be cleaned and watched carefully, because radiation tends to cause decay, eventually necessitating crown amputation and even causing bone necrosis.

Because Mr. Long has a habit of neglecting his teeth, teach him proper mouth care and urge him to rinse his mouth with a saline or peroxide solution five to ten times a day after treatments begin. The dentist will give him a topical fluoride to apply to his teeth for 5 minutes after brushing and outfit him with a protective fluoride carrier that will cover his teeth during radiation.

INDEX

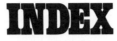